RELATIONSHIPS IN OLD AGE

THE GUILFORD SERIES ON PERSONAL RELATIONSHIPS

Steve Duck, *Editor*

Department of Communication Studies
The University of Iowa

Relationships in Old Age:
Coping with the Challenge of Transition
Robert O. Hansson
Bruce N. Carpenter

Friendships Between Women
Pat O'Connor

Conflicts in Intimate Relationships
Dudley D. Cahn

Relationships in Old Age

Coping with the Challenge of Transition

Robert O. Hansson
Bruce N. Carpenter

THE GUILFORD PRESS
New York London

©1994   The Guilford Press
A Division of Guilford Publications, Inc.
72 Spring Street, New York, NY 10012

Printed in the United States of America

This book is printed on acid-free paper.

Last digit is print number: 9   8   7   6   5   4   3   2   1

Library of Congress Cataloging-in-Publication Data

Hansson, Robert, O.,
    Relationships in old age : coping with the challenge of transition
/ Robert O. Hansson, Bruce N. Carpenter.
        p.   cm. — (Guilford series on personal relationships)
    Includes bibliographical references and index.
    ISBN 0-89862-198-4
    1. Aged — Social networks. 2. Aged — Psychology. 3. Interpersonal
relations. 4. Intergenerational relations. I. Carpenter, Bruce N.
II. Title. III. Series.
    [DNLM: 1. Interpersonal Relations — in old age. 2. Aged —
psychology. 3. Aging — physiology. 3. Social Environment. WT 30
H251r 1994]
HQ1061.H337   1994
305.26 — dc20
DNLM/DLC
for Library of Congress   93-46488
                                                                   CIP

I dedicate this book to two individuals: to my wife, Kathleen, whose patience, love, and support have made the difference during the most important moments of my life; and to my sister, Maggie, whose devotion and care for our mother during the last years of her life enriched us all.

R.O.H.

I dedicate this book to my parents, A. J. and Lorna Carpenter, who taught me the good things about families and relationships, and who continue to teach me about successful aging.

B.N.C.

Acknowledgments

A book such as this is in part a product of those who went before. Gerontologists and researchers from the broad field of personal relationships have advanced considerably our understanding of the social environments of older adults. We sincerely acknowledge the contributions of the many scientists whose work we have cited in this volume.

We wish to express our thanks, also, to a number of persons to whom we are especially indebted. It was our pleasure for many years to collaborate with Warren Jones on the topic of relational competence; many of the earliest and most insightful ideas were his. Steven Hobfoll and Mary Ann Parris Stephens encouraged us early on (for a conference at the Kent State Forum) to think specifically about the connections between relational competence and stress in aging families. Similarly, Steve Duck, our editor on this project, provided feedback that helped immensely in shaping the final product. Finally, we thank Julie Hansson for her extremely helpful editorial assistance with large portions of the manuscript.

Preface

Later life is a time of critical transitions. The aging experience demands continual adaptation to changing physical, psychological, and social capacities, and to the implications of these changes for one's economic status, independence, and life satisfaction. Fortunately, most older adults find that their family and social relationships can be an important source of support at such times.

Researchers have learned much about these support processes, and about the kinds of interactions, exchanges, relationships, and family systems involved. However, less attention has been paid to the role of the older adult as an active player in the process, one capable to some degree of initiating and enhancing potentially supportive personal relationships. Such competence on the part of older adults would seem especially important, since the personal relationships upon which long-term social support depends are themselves often problematic.

The focus of this book, then, is on what the *individual* brings to the situation that could change the odds of successfully constructing, accessing, or maintaining potentially supportive personal relationships. Our own research in this area has focused on *relational competence,* a construct encompassing temperamental, cognitive, and emotional characteristics, and social competencies that are likely to be valuable in the process.

The first five chapters of the book establish the context in which relational competence becomes important for older adults. The reader is introduced early on to the nature of aging, to the experience of loss, decline, and adaptation, to models of coping and adaptation available in the gerontological literature, and to how interpersonal resources can influence coping and adaptation. Another theme introduced early in the book concerns the critical role of relationships in old age. Old age is a time when significant relationships are lost through the death of friends and loved ones. Beyond that, however, personal relationships can be important sources of logistical, social, and psychological support, but they can also be sources of conflict, tension, and stress. We devote considerable space to the problematic side of support relationships in later life.

In Chapter 5, we propose a model of the Interpersonal Contexts of Old Age. Gerontological researchers have made considerable progress in mapping the interpersonal settings in which elderly persons must function (friendships, family, caregiver networks, the workplace, congregate housing, institutions, etc.). The proposed model permits an integrative analysis of the many categories of interpersonal settings with respect to the coping or adaptational demands they place on older adults. It also sets the stage for a parallel analysis of relational competence.

The latter half of the book is devoted to the construct of relational competence, to its components and how they can be measured, and to social and clinical interventions that might be guided by the approach. We introduce our model of relational competence, the interpersonal characteristics it encompasses, and the functions they serve in two general domains (the *initiation* and *enhancement* of important relationships). We also review research on the manner in which relational competence shapes and influences the quality of our relationships, and enhances functioning in other areas of our lives (e.g., health or occupational behavior).

The final two chapters explore the potential of social and clinical interventions for enhancing an older person's social functioning and personal coping resources. Such interventions range from the enhancement of naturally occurring social processes (e.g., within care environments, families, or community institutions) to more directive counseling interventions (e.g., to promote social skills, provide insight, or construct coping mechanisms).

The book is intended for advanced undergraduates, graduate students, researchers, and practitioners. We examine recent research from many disciplines (e.g., Gerontology, Psychology, Sociology, Family Relations, Personal Relationships, Communications, Nursing, and Social Work), synthesizing and integrating each discipline as it relates to the topic of the book. In doing so, we address the implications for application, practice, and future research.

At the same time, it is our intention to tell the story of older adults and their relationships in a wide variety of interpersonal settings. In this effort, we hope to introduce the student reader to the multidisciplinary nature of gerontological studies and to how our understanding of the lives of aging adults can be enhanced by the broader view.

Contents

CHAPTER 1

THE CRITICAL ROLE OF RELATIONSHIPS

The aging experience is complex. As early as middle adulthood (e.g., ages 35–60 years), we begin to encounter physiological, psychological, and social changes associated with growing older. These changes are typically quite gradual, however, and within a person's range of adaptation. Our primary focus in this book concerns the more difficult years of older adulthood.

The term "older adult" generally refers to people over the age of 60 years. It is often useful, however, to make finer distinctions even within this age group. We are now living longer and healthier lives. Many older people do not experience serious illness or disability until their early 70s, and so they do not feel old or identify as being old until faced with such an incident. These individuals are often called the "young-old." The "old-old" (ages 75–85 years) and the "very old" (85+ years) comprise the fastest growing segments of the American population, and researchers have just begun to understand the nature of their experience.

Later life also reflects considerable individual diversity. Some persons exhibit health or cognitive declines quite early, whereas others continue to function as well or better than ever in many of the domains of their lives into their 80s and 90s. Gerontologists now argue that any early declines probably reflect pathology, rather than the effects of aging. At some point in every life, however, age-related losses accumulate and may produce a crisis. At such times, personal relationships and the support of family and friends can become critical to an older adult's adaptation and well-being.

We will be focusing throughout this book on the functions that relationships serve in the lives of older adults. We will be moving quickly to analyses of these relationships and the social care systems that support older persons in coping with age-related change. The reader will note, however, that the experience of aging often requires our personal relationships, families, and community support networks also to evolve and adapt. Often this goes well; sometimes it does not.

Many of the relationships issues important to older adults are also relevant (and have been studied extensively) across the life-span. In the first part of this chapter, we briefly review a number of fundamental themes from this broader literature (e.g., the role of relationships in health, well-being, and successful life functioning). The second part of the chapter then introduces the relationship issues that arise in old age.

POSITIVE RELATIONSHIPS AS A DESIRED OUTCOME

We should begin our discussion by noting that close and effective relationships are desirable in and of themselves. Social functioning is integral to human functioning, not only because it leads to other desired outcomes, but because we crave and need contact with others.

We are social creatures, and extended loss of social contact typically leads to unhappiness and dysfunction. It is well established, for example, that depriving infants and young children of the contact associated with good mothering leads to developmental delays and maladjustment, even when physical needs are well met (e.g., Tizard & Tizard, 1970). Similarly, observers have long noted that the loss of important relationships leads to feelings of emptiness and depression (Freud, 1917/1957; Bowlby, 1980).

Persons involved with positive relationships tend to be less affected by everyday problems, to be more effective, and to act with a greater sense of control and independence. Those without relationships often become isolated, cynical, mistrusting, and depressed. Those caught in poor relationships tend to develop and maintain negative perceptions of self, find life less satisfying, and often lack the skills or motivation to make changes (Duck, 1988a). Indeed, the power of relationships is reflected in the tendency for some in negative relationships to stay in them; they often report a fear of having no relationships and consider a bad one better than none at all (Davis & Hagen, 1992).

Relationships influence our lives in so many ways and sometimes so subtly that we scarcely notice. In many respects, our established relationships are the anchors around which we structure our immediate and life-long priorities, our daily schedules and significant events, and our views of self and the world. To remove relationships would remove much of the reason for our actions, spanning our most mundane to our most unusual behaviors.

IMPORTANT CONSEQUENCES OF RELATIONSHIPS AND SOCIAL FUNCTIONING

In spite of their fundamental nature, researchers have come to understand the role of relationships, in part, by studying their consequences. In the following pages we describe two of the more general consequences of social functioning: well-being and health. First, however, it is useful to consider some ways in which the various consequences are organized.

Benefits and Costs

Much of the study of relational benefits has focused on social support. Social support has been defined in a variety of ways, but it typically refers to the presence of a supportive network or to the supportive actions, attitudes, and emotional climate provided by others. Some forms of social support can be provided by most anyone, including professionals, community agency workers, and even strangers. However, most social support derives from those with whom one has an enduring relationship, primarily family and friends.

Three types of social support are often described (e.g., Cohen & McKay, 1984; Schaefer, Coyne, & Lazarus, 1981), each referring to a different kind of benefit. *Instrumental support* refers to the tangible benefits of a supportive relationship. For example, giving money and other physical resources is instrumental support, but so is solving a problem for someone or providing access to another person who can help. *Informational support* involves sharing of knowledge. Thus, one might provide new information, offer opinions, or help someone think through a problem or consider alternatives. *Emotional support* refers to the sense of belonging and value that comes from perceiving others as caring and willing to give of self for you. Rather than directly helping to solve problems, emotional support seems to promote resiliency and positive ways of thinking about oneself and one's situation.

Social support, however, is not identical to what we mean by relationships. An alternative model that focuses more on relationships is provided by Weiss (1974; Cutrona & Russell, 1987), who described a set of six "social provisions." *Attachment* refers to emotional closeness, yielding a sense of security. *Social integration* involves shared interests and activities, so that one feels a part of a group. *Reassur-*

ance of worth is feedback that one is valued because of personal attributes. *Reliable alliance* is the recognition that others are available to help in time of need. *Guidance* is information and advice offered by others. Finally, *opportunity for nurturance* reflects being valued in a relationship for what one does for one's partners, specifically that others depend on one for their own well-being.

Relationships do not lead only to benefits. They may also involve significant costs, although in positive relationships unnecessary costs are avoided or minimized and benefits outweigh costs in the long run. Researchers have recently attempted to delineate the detrimental functions of relationships (e.g., Rook & Pietromonaco, 1987), but there is less theoretical work. We propose three types of costs to illustrate the principle.

First, relationships can place *instrumental demands* upon partners. Typically, one is expected to spend time with and do things for the partner, such as sharing income or maintaining a home. One reason we adopt roles in relationships is to reduce overall costs by making this exchange of instrumental benefits more efficient. Compartmentalization of responsibilities often accomplishes this—for some tasks one can perform the task for a group more efficiently than if each group member must perform the task for him/herself. A second cost is *emotional vulnerability.* Intimacy, or even familiarity, exposes one to intentional or unintentional hurt from the partner, such as through dependency, attachment that makes loss more damaging, manipulation, or betrayal. Finally, *compromise,* although necessary to social adaptation, requires relational partners to adjust or give up personal goals and alter behavior in nonpreferred ways.

Well-Being

Much of what we get out of relationships benefits our psychological and emotional well-being. By well-being we mean a variety of things, including happiness, life satisfaction, a positive sense of self, and relative freedom from negative mood states or psychopathology. Many people prefer being with a friend when engaging in pleasant activities, such as going to a movie. Social events are, for most of us, enjoyable. We depend on feedback from others for development of our self-concept and validation of our self-worth. It even seems true that relational functioning at times has the power to color the whole sense of one's life. For example, severe marital discord is highly disruptive and often plunges whole families into depression and dysfunctional behavior patterns (e.g., Gable, Belsky, & Crnic, 1992; Reid & Crisafulli, 1990).

Interestingly, because of the close connections between well-being and positive relational functioning, measures of social satisfaction (such as loneliness; e.g., Russell, Peplau, & Cutrona, 1980) are sometimes used as indices of well-being. Similarly, measures of anxiety, depression, and self-esteem often include items inquiring about relational satisfaction or one's sense of being valued and appreciated by others. Social indices, such as social support, number of friendships, and loneliness, are typically found to be highly correlated with measures of self-esteem, depression, anxiety, and optimism.

At least as far back as Freud (1917/1957), the connections between depression and relationships have been postulated and verified. The focus varies—from loss of a relationship, to relationship problems and relational stress, to how relationships block or offset the ability of negative events to evoke depression—but the importance of relationships is clear. This tie to relationships may be observed in other forms of psychopathology as well. For example, Monroe (1990) found substantial negative correlations between marital satisfaction and scores on several personality disorder dimensions (including borderline, avoidant, dependent, paranoid, schizoid, and antisocial personality). This association is reflected in the diagnostic criteria of many psychiatric disorders, especially including the personality disorders (American Psychiatric Association, 1987). Extending these ideas, Horowitz and Vitkus (1986) proposed a model of how relational dysfunction underlies much psychological distress and contributes to various psychiatric disorders.

Health and Illness

Relationships also appear to impact life systems seemingly far removed from social functioning. One of the most intriguing and well-studied domains is that of health and illness. Relationship variables have been found to be associated with a wide variety of health outcomes, usually with the finding that positive social functioning leads to better health, and relational difficulties contribute to illness. Although we are often unable to say with certainty that social functioning *causes* these health outcomes, evidence is accruing to support that conclusion. In its 1991 report *Healthy People 2000,* the U.S. Department of Health and Human Services set forth national health objectives to be met by the year 2000. Of particular interest, the report concluded that social isolation is a major risk factor for functional difficulties in older persons, and it encourages community networks to help older adults maintain independence.

The list of relevant associations between health and social functioning is long and varied. For example, loss of relationships, especially bereavement following death of a family member, is predictive of one's own morbidity and mortality (Berkman & Breslow, 1983; House, Landis, & Umberson, 1988; Stroebe & Stroebe, 1993). Interestingly, Silverstein and Bengtson (1991) found that close parent–child relations reduced the mortality rate of recently widowed older persons. Similarly, those with weak social networks appear several times more likely to die within a given time period than those with strong networks (e.g., Berkman, 1985).

A variety of studies have found that effective social functioning is associated with better immune functioning. This is important because as immune functioning is suppressed, the likelihood of disease is increased. For example, lower immune functioning was found in lonely medical students (Kiecolt-Glaser, Garner, et al., 1984), and elderly women reporting good social interaction had better immune functioning than did those with poor interaction (Thomas, Goodwin, & Goodwin, 1985). Animal studies suggest that emotional states (e.g., depression) associated with loss and separation lead to an increase in glucocorticoids, hormones which suppress immune functioning (Laudenslager, 1988). Similarly, social support in humans is negatively correlated with stress hormone levels (Kiecolt-Glaser, Ricker, et al., 1984). The interested reader is referred to Laudenslager (1988) and to Irwin and Pike (1993) for excellent overviews of recent research on social loss and immune functioning.

Similar associations have been found for cancer survival (Waxler-Morrison, Hislop, Mears, & Can, 1991), heart disease (see Chapter 7), and general health in poor, frail elderly (Mor-Barak, Miller, & Syme, 1991). Sometimes the magnitude of the associations is large enough to place the social factor on a level with other factors known to increase risk for disease. For example, this appears to be the case when we consider social support and relational functioning in comparison with known risk factors for cardiovascular disease, such as smoking (Atkins, Kaplan, & Toshima, 1991).

MECHANISMS BY WHICH RELATIONSHIPS IMPACT LIFE FUNCTIONING

The interplay between relationships and various domains of life functioning is complex. For example, the usefulness of social support for dealing with illness has been shown repeatedly; but illness itself, especially chronic illness (which is common among the elderly), interferes with relationships and encourages social isolation. Simply resisting the isolating effects of age-related declines, losses, and illness may be an important form of coping with old age.

There are two prominent models of how relationships and social support impact outcomes (e.g., Cohen & Syme, 1985). The first, the *stress-buffering hypothesis,* suggests that negative outcomes are a result of stress (life change, negative events, excessive demands for coping). Under this hypothesis, social support operates mainly to reduce — or buffer — the negative impact of stress. This view suggests that persons not currently experiencing stress receive little or no benefit from relationships. But such a hypothesis helps explain why the areas of life functioning impacted by relationships are much the same as those impacted by stress. Those with support, according to this hypothesis, are presumed to have more help for meeting demands and to feel better about themselves so that demands are perceived as less threatening. For example, a loving, positive relationship likely impacts the way one reacts to failure experiences (e.g., "How can I be bad or be a failure if this person loves me?").

The second model, termed the *main-effects model,* postulates that stress is only one variable that leads to negative outcomes. Social functioning is simply a separate variable promoting positive outcomes. The main-effects model suggests that a positive social environment encourages health and well-being whether or not stress is present. For example, relationships probably impact the attitude with which one approaches life; without relationships one might be more tenuous in self-concept and more dependent on external validation, resulting in greater anxiety or self-doubt. This could contribute to negative outcomes, whether or not stress was present.

Studies have often suggested that one or the other of these models is more powerful for explaining a particular outcome. However, substantial evidence exists in support of both the stress-buffering and the main-effects models (e.g., Cohen & Syme, 1985; Kaplan, Sallis, & Patterson, 1993; Kaplan & Toshima, 1990). Apparently, the nature of support, stressors, and other factors affect the way in which social functioning impacts various outcomes.

Given the complexities of relationships, there are probably other, indirect ways in which relationships impact life functioning. For example, relationships may have a greater impact on health habits than on actual health. Family and friends may encourage us to practice health-promoting behaviors. Perhaps for similar reasons, people benefit more from weight loss programs when they participate with a friend (Dubbert & Wilson, 1984). Also, family members may be more inclined to cook well-balanced meals when they feel responsible for another's welfare. Alternatively, the disruption of relational patterns can undermine health-promoting behaviors. For example, Rosenbloom and Whittington (1993) found that becoming widowed changed substantially the social environment of mealtimes. Elderly widows (compared to a control sample of married women) found meals significantly less enjoyable, were more likely to eat alone, and sustained less adequate levels of nutrient intake. Notably, widows who continued to experience grief-related distress were particularly likely to have counter productive eating habits and less adequate nutrition.

Finally, personal relationships are multifaceted, sometimes yielding unexpected results. For example, Barrera and Baca (1990) found that one's reaction to offered support depends on other factors, such as the conflictual nature of the relationship. It would not be surprising, then, to expect some acts to be interpreted as supportive by some and meddling by others. Thus, we might take advice better from a professional than a family member. Similarly, there needs to be some match between needs and what the relationship has to offer. Validation of self-worth might come best from intimate others, but following a natural disaster, financial aid might be most needed. We deal with these subtleties at some length in Chapters 3, 4, and 5.

RELATIONSHIP ISSUES AND OUTCOMES IN OLD AGE

We have seen from the above discussion how personal relationships can enhance life functioning generally. These processes are particularly critical for the elderly. For example, an older person's relational ties and support networks can play a central role in the decision to retire (Ekerdt, 1989; Fletcher & Hansson, 1991) or to seek supportive housing arrangements (Lawton, 1980). They can also facilitate adaptive health behavior and the effective utilization of health services (Shanas & Maddox, 1985). It should not be a surprise, therefore, that health care practitioners would consider their older patients' support relationships in trying to meet their diverse needs without encouraging premature dependency or causing undue economic burden on society. Similarly, an understanding of older persons' support relationships can be useful in formulating social and economic policy, for example, in considering eligibility for subsidized services or public housing.

Both researchers and policy makers have shown much interest in the relationships of the elderly. We introduce here a sampling of this informative research to establish a context for much of the discussion to follow.

Relationships serve a wide variety of positive functions among older adults. These range from instrumental assistance (with finances, housing, or transportation) to an array of social and psychological supports (House, 1981; Thoits, 1982; Weiss, 1974). As we shall see below, the provision of instrumental support is increasingly important among older persons. Social and psychological supports available from close relatives and friends tend to center around acceptance, respect, compatibility, warmth, and sharing. The functions of broader networks of family and friends are more likely to involve attention and inclusion, affection, assistance, and intimacy (Lawton & Moss, 1987).

HEALTH ISSUES

The importance of family support becomes even more evident when we consider the changing nature of health experience in old age. Although individuals may vary, the later years are a time of progressive, chronic loss in physiological functioning. Predictable, age-related changes have been noted, for example, in the immune and pulmonary systems, in the ability to perform the activities of daily living (e.g., cooking, cleaning, self-care), and in the body's capacity to recover from such traumatic events as surgery, falls, or acute illness (Rowe, 1985).

Nor do the dramatic increases in life expectancy in recent decades necessarily mean more years of functional independence. For example, adults currently 65 to 69 years of age have a life expectancy of some 16.5 years, but 6.5 years of that time will likely involve considerable loss of function (Katz et al., 1983). Table 1.1 shows the increasing incidence in old age of a wide variety of chronic health conditions. It should also be noted that an older person may be experiencing several of these conditions concurrently. Table 1.2 shows how chronic health conditions translate into functional limitations and eventual threats to an older adult's capacity for independent living. By the mid- to late 70s, for example, over 20% have difficulty walk-

TABLE 1.1. Percentage of Older Persons with Selected Chronic Health Conditions (1987)

Chronic condition	Ages 65–74 (%)	Ages 75 and older (%)
Arthritis	46.4	51.2
Hypertension	39.2	33.7
Heart condition	28.5	32.2
Hearing impairment	26.4	34.8
Orthopedic impairment	15.5	18.2
Diabetes	9.8	9.8
Visual impairment	5.6	11.1

Source: U.S. Bureau of the Census. (1990). *Statistical Abstract of the United States: 1990* (110th ed., p. 118, Table 190). Washington, DC: U.S. Government Printing Office.

TABLE 1.2. Percentage of Older Persons with Selected Functional Limitations (1984)

Limitation	Ages 65–74 (%)	Ages 75–84 (%)	(%) 85+ yr.
Walking	14.2	22.9	39.9
Getting outside	5.6	12.3	31.3
Bathing	6.4	12.3	27.9
Dressing	4.3	7.6	16.6
Preparing meals	4.0	8.8	26.1
Shopping	6.4	15.0	37.0
Managing money	2.2	6.3	24.0
Doing heavy housework	18.6	28.7	47.8

Source: U.S. Bureau of the Census. (1990). *Statistical Abstract of the United States: 1990* (110th ed., p. 120, Table 193). Washington, DC: U.S. Government Printing Office.

ing and doing housework. By the mid-80s those percentages appear to double, and large numbers also begin to have difficulty with self-sustaining tasks such as bathing, dressing, and preparing meals. These trends, then, suggest an increasing dependency at some point in one's old age on family and on more formal health services.

The nature of the illness experience also becomes more complex in later life. Older adults are more likely to be suffering from multiple diseases or disabilities and to be taking a greater number and variety of prescribed medications. Symptoms are often internal and nonspecific to a given organ system, thus difficult to diagnose and treat. Physical and mental health are also significantly interrelated among older persons. For example, increasing physical distress or disability is likely to be accompanied by depressive symptoms. Mental health problems, on the other hand, may interfere with recognition or management of physical disorders (Cohen, 1990; Gatz & Smyer, 1992). Added to such complexity is the tendency of older persons to underreport health symptoms, often because they believe such symptoms to reflect the "normal" and inevitable problems of aging, because they fear painful or costly hospitalization, or because of cognitive impairment (Rowe, 1985).

It is clear that the well-being of many older people will eventually depend on the ability of the family to provide not only psychological and social support, but also case-management or caregiving services (Brody, 1985; Cantor, 1991; Cantor & Little, 1985; Eyde & Rich, 1983). This dependency becomes most salient in the face of crisis (such as a major disabling health event). A recent study of older persons who had experienced a hip fracture illustrates the point. In this study, the most frequent coping strategy was found to be the seeking of social support (Roberto, 1992).

Unfortunately, the family and friendship networks of some older persons in this situation are either smaller or less emotionally supportive. These individuals are faced with having to seek help from alternative sources. They are therefore more likely to be found among applicants to public social service agencies (Auslander & Litwin, 1990).

Gerontologists have generally concluded that the size and availability of family support networks are the two most important factors in deferring or preventing the institutionalization of elderly persons (e.g., Hickey, 1980; Lawton, 1981). Furthermore, active social involvements (e.g., visiting and talking with friends) that are made possible by integration into a social network are also associated with a decreased risk of institutionalization and mortality, even after controlling for age, sex, and perceived health status (Steinbach, 1992). In contrast, living alone and widowhood are associated with increased risks of institutionalization (Wolinsky & Johnson, 1992).

LIVING ARRANGEMENTS AND SOCIAL INTEGRATION OF OLDER ADULTS

Most older adults are not socially isolated. However, their living arrangements and degree of integration into supportive family structures are quite diverse. Of those aged 65 and over, 67% live with family. This percentage decreases with age. Approximately 13% live with relatives other than a spouse, and 2% live with nonrelatives. About 30% live alone (U.S. Bureau of the Census, 1990). As may be seen in Table 1.3, however, these figures differ considerably by gender and race. That is, women and blacks in the United States are less likely to be living with a spouse after age 65. White women not living with a spouse are more likely to live alone. However, black women not living with a

TABLE 1.3. Living Arrangements by Race and Sex of Persons 65 Years and Older (1988)

	All races[a]		White		Black	
% living	%M	%F	%M	%F	%M	%F
Alone	16.2	40.6	15.4	41.1	26.4	38.5
With spouse	75.1	39.9	76.2	41.0	62.5	27.1
With other relatives	6.7	17.2	6.4	15.6	8.6	30.8

[a]Includes other races not shown separately.
Source: U.S. Bureau of the Census. (1990). *Statistical Abstract of the United States: 1990* (110th ed., p. 49, Table 62). Washington, DC: U.S. Government Printing Office.

spouse are nearly as likely to be living with other relatives as living alone.

Approximately 80% of American adults aged 65 or over have living children. Two-thirds of the children live within 30 minutes of the older parent. Over 60% of older adults have been found to have weekly visits with their children, and 75% visit by telephone at least weekly. Some older persons, however, will have had to enter congregate housing, shared housing, or institutions (American Association of Retired Persons, 1990). This, of course, entails entering a new social system and new (hopefully supportive) relationships.

Older persons are highly diverse with regard to their level of dependency on supportive personal relationships. That is, they differ widely in health status, economic security, and other personal coping resources (Kingson, Hirshorn, & Cornman, 1986). However, families do remain an important source of support and health-related care for older persons. Such support can considerably diminish the consequences of disease, and it is a critical consideration in decisions about institutionalization. Indeed, for every older person who resides in a nursing home, two similarly impaired persons are able to live at home (Rowe, 1985). The provision of support often tends to be reciprocal, with older family members sharing financial personal resources with their children well into the children's middle-adulthood (e.g., help with mortgages, grandchildren's education, baby-sitting, housekeeping, and the like; cf. Kingson et al., 1986). With increasing age, however, adult children and extended kin networks experience a growing awareness of the roles they will need to assume in providing more direct and sustained support or intervention (e.g., Brody, 1985; Cantor, 1991; Cantor & Little, 1985; Hansson, Nelson, et al., 1990; Shanas, 1979; Sussman, 1985).

Cantor (1979, 1991) proposed that families, communities, and more formal institutions typically interact as an integrated system of "social care" for older adults in need. She likened this system to a series of overlapping concentric circles, each representing a distinct level and form of support. The older individual is at the center of the system. Family members, neighbors and kin, community and government agencies, respectively, occupy circles further from the center. The social care system is viewed initially to augment individual mastery and coping efforts on the part of older persons. But it provides psychological support, assistance with the activities of daily living, and more advanced care in time of illness and disability. The system is dynamic, with support resources responding to changes in the older adult's changing status (and to the changing potential of family and kin to provide support). Older people typically prefer to move outward in the model, toward more formal support resources, only when the limits of the family and informal supports have been reached.

A number of recent trends in American family life, however, could seriously impact the family's participation in providing such support (Cantor, 1991). For example:

1. Multigeneration families are becoming common.
2. With a declining birth rate and increased longevity, families are becoming more vertical, with a greater generational span and fewer siblings in younger generations to provide support.
3. Increased life expectancies mean that adult caregivers may spend a longer period of years caring for their parents than for their children.
4. Continuity of care for older family members is becoming more complex with dramatic increases in divorce, reconstructed, and single-parent families, increasing numbers of women entering the workforce, and geographic mobility within families.
5. With improved health care and longevity, the onset of age-related disability is increasingly being deferred until later in life. The role of family caregiver is therefore being assumed at a later age, when the caregiver also may be more vulnerable physically or financially.

Trends in longevity, changes in the nature of the health experience in old age, and changes in the American family structure have thus combined to produce what Brody (1985) has called "parent care as a normative family stress" (p. 19). Current research on the implications of such family stress for the care of older family members will be reviewed in Chapter 4. In addition, a number of age-related changes may have implications for the development and maintenance of mutually supportive friendships in old age. Life events such as retirement, health crises, widowhood, deaths of old friends, involuntary relocation, and the like may result in narrower friendship networks or may restrict social participation and the occupation of former social roles. Diminished income, health, or independence may result in an inability to maintain reciprocity in friendships, and eventual withdrawal from these relationships (Allen & Adams, 1989; Blieszner, 1989).

As the challenges evolve, family and community support structures will likely adapt. An important example of such adaptation (and diversity of response) is provided by extended family networks in the African-American community. Such networks often include "alternative family members" (or "fictive kin") in addition to blood kin; these are friends whose relationships assume the affectional ties, rights, and responsibilities of biological family (Johnson & Barer, 1990, p. 730). Fictive kin may be drawn from informal or formal associations (e.g., church, shared households, foster-parent or grandparent relationships, home care workers). Research suggests that extended family networks of this type can be flexible and rich sources of support for all members, including the elderly. They have played an important role in the ability of the black community to cope with economic distress, discrimination, and resulting instability (Johnson & Barer, 1990; Stack, 1975; Sussman, 1985; Willie, 1988).

CHAPTER 2

ADAPTATION AND COPING IN THE AGING CONTEXT

G erontologists now know a great deal about age-related change in humans. Longitudinal studies, following the same individuals over long periods of time, have examined the average trajectory of such change with some precision in many areas of physiological function, physical and emotional health, cognitive status, and personality. This body of research has provided a useful picture of those areas in which significant age-related change should be expected and those in which it should not.

One of the most important lessons from this research, however, is that a unit of change on any of these measures of status in later life does not necessarily translate uniformly into diminished functional competence or quality of life. That is, identical declines in vision, hearing, cardiac function, or memory may have very different implications for differing individuals. We shall see, in this chapter, that many factors can mediate (compound or inhibit) the consequences of age-related deficits. Such factors include genetic background, concurrent age-related changes the individual may be experiencing, and available social and economic coping resources. Perhaps most important, however, are the personal coping resources the individual brings to the situation (e.g., personality, skill, maturity, perspective, motivation, experience).

It should not be a surprise, therefore, that any assessment of an older adult's ability to function (e.g., after a significant health event or hospitalization) would need to take many factors into account. That is, it would probably be important to assess not only physical and mental status but also one's motivation to regain function and independence and the supportive potential of the physical and social environment to which the individual wishes to return (Kane & Kane, 1981).

Our primary focus in this volume is the role of supportive personal relationships. We explore throughout the book the many ways in which relationships influence adaptation and coping in old age. To set the context, however, in this chapter we provide a brief overview of the nature of age-related decline and loss in the later years. In addition, we review several of the dominant theories of adaptation, coping, and successful aging from the gerontological literature.

AGE-RELATED DECLINE AND LOSS

Physiological Capacity

We noted in Chapter 1 the changing nature of health experience in later life, with its increased emphasis on progressive, chronic illness and increasing levels of functional limitation. However, researchers have also been able to provide estimates of the rate of decline in important physiological capacities across the life-span. As body composition changes and organ systems deteriorate, functional capacities such as neural conduction, metabolic rate, cardiac output, filtration, lung capacity, plasma flow, and the immune response all decline (Rowe, 1977, 1985). The interactive effects of such declines (with each other and with disease process) can dramatically undermine the organism's homeostatic capacity. The result is a diminished ability with age to recover from acute trauma, for example, from accidents, burns, illness, surgical procedures, or intensive medication (Feller, Flora, & Bawol, 1976; Rowe, 1985).

Cognitive Capacity

Longitudinal data are now also available with which to estimate the nature of cognitive change in later life. The Seattle Longitudinal Study, for example, assessed five primary abilities (verbal meaning, spatial orientation, inductive reasoning, number, and word fluency) every 7 years (Schaie, 1983, 1990a). This study has provided several important insights over the years regarding cognitive changes in adulthood. Perhaps the most important overall finding, however, was that we should not expect significant, age-related deficits until the mid- to late 60s. Individuals exhibiting earlier declines should be assessed for the presence of pathology. The different cognitive abilities appear to follow varying trajectories with respect to the age in adulthood at which peak performance is reached, the age at which significant declines become evident, and subsequent rates of decline. In the late 60s, gradual declines in performance begin to appear, first in those abilities involving speed of performance or abstract reasoning (Willis, 1985).

Recent analyses from the Seattle Study data have focused on the reverse side of previously reported patterns. For example, Schaie (1990b) examined the proportion of individuals at ages 60, 67, 74, and 81 who had *not* declined in each of the abilities over the preceding 7-year period. Results indicated that at age 60, 75%–85% of subjects had maintained or improved function depending on the specific abilities. Even at age 81, over 60% of subjects retained previous levels of function on all abilities (Schaie, 1990b). Age-related declines that did occur, however, appeared to be ability-specific rather than global ones. That is, among all age groups, nearly 100% of subjects retained previous level of function on at least one ability. Depending on age, 15%–40% of subjects successfully retained function on all five abilities (Schaie, 1990b).

Changes in Economic Status

As a group, persons over age 65 have actually increased their economic well-being in recent decades (U.S. Bureau of the Census, 1988). Much of that improvement has reflected automatic price indexing of pension benefits and the manner in which the over-65 population is changing, (i.e., newly turned 65-year-olds, on average, have greater incomes and accrued wealth than do those older persons who die each year (Smeeding, 1990).

It can be misleading, however, to analyze the economic circumstances of the older population in such broad terms. The story is in individual and group differences. For example, the very old and single women living alone remain at considerable economic risk. In 1986, the percentages of widows aged 65–74, 75–84, and 85 + who fell below the poverty line were 19.8%, 20.3%, and 23.4%, respectively. This compared to a rate of 12.6% for all persons aged 65 + (U.S. Congress, House Ways and Means Committee, 1988). Similarly, the likelihood of older people falling below the poverty line differs by race, with the percentages of white, black, and Hispanic persons aged 65 and over who fell below the poverty line in 1988 being 10.0%, 32.2%, and 22.4%, respectively (U.S. Bureau of the Census, 1990, Table 745). Drawing the circle a little larger, to include the officially poor and near-poor (near-poor criterion = 125% of poverty line), 20.3% of all elderly and 35.2% of elderly female householders with no spouse present were classified as poor or near-poor (U.S. Bureau of the Census, 1988).

Social Stress

Old age is not generally experienced as a time of social isolation or loneliness. However, we described in Chapter 1 how age-related circumstances (e.g., involving health, finances, or retirement) can begin to restrict social interaction. As we discuss in Chapters 3 and 4, a variety of additional factors can further constrain the meaningful social involvement of older persons. Such factors include the loss of friends and family through death, stereotypic treatment of the elderly, the contraction of social roles (e.g., parenting) in later years, and the stressful effects of an older person's growing frailty and dependency on family relationships.

Implications

The research findings discussed above raise some very interesting questions regarding the development of health, social, and economic policy. Of particular concern are our basic assumptions about the outlook for a society's aged members. For example:

- How useful are observed average patterns of age-related change and decline in devising strategies for health care, social policy, employment, and retirement policy?
- Is there an underlying order to adult development, involving universal stages through which we all must eventually pass? Or is development less orderly and predictable, reflecting in each individual a unique mix of interacting influences?
- Should a deterministic (and generally pessimistic) view prevail regarding the aging process, normative patterns of expected decline, and diminished competence or ability to productively contribute to society?
- What are the place and potential of the elderly in a society?
- Are there circumstances under which some individuals age more successfully than most, and what can be learned from those who age more successfully?
- How shall we treat individual differences in the aging process?

THE NATURE OF ADULT DEVELOPMENT

Integrating our knowledge about the nature of aging has often been difficult, given the multidisciplinary nature of the field. The questions asked, methodologies used, and conclusions drawn by gerontological researchers reflect immensely diverse perspectives. Nevertheless, a number of theoretical models have emerged to guide our thinking about the nature of adult development. The underlying assumptions of each model provide important clues for understanding developmental change in later life and for understanding the experience of age-related stress, adaptation, and coping. Three theoretical approaches, in particular, have taken positions regarding the universality of the aging experience and the utility of normative models for predicted decline in function.

The Seasons of Life

Life-stage models are perhaps best represented by Levinson's (1978, 1986) broadly integrative model of adult development. Levinson's analyses of adult development rested initially on several assumptions. First, it was important to think about development in terms of one's personal life course, to obtain a sense for the continuity and history of an individual's life and why it had unfolded as it had. Simultaneously, however, it was important to view one's development in the context of the human life cycle, to understand the influence of age-related changes, choices, relational patterns, and vulnerabilities common to us all. Finally, it was important to obtain an integrated picture of the individual's current life structure, that is, what one's life is like now. The life structure would therefore incorporate all the important elements of one's life, from the objective aspects of occupational and relationship involvements to subjective aspirations, satisfactions, frustrations, and so on.

Levinson conducted extensive biographical interviews with his research subjects in order to explore these issues. He mapped out what appeared to be the major developmental periods of the life cycle and the tasks, relational patterns, and psychological characteristics that appeared to be associated with each. During each stage, and during the transition periods separating the stages, individuals were viewed to face serious (often threatening) challenges, choices, demands for new commitments, and the need come to terms with a "new me." The focus, then, was on the evolving self in response to the demands of succeeding life stages. Of particular concern in this process was the identification of important areas of continuity, change, and qualitative development.

In this context, the period of late adulthood (age 60 and over) was considered to have been shaped in large part by a growing need to cope with physical decline, chronic illness, diminished vigor and competence, and reduced involvement in social and work roles. The model acknowledges that individuals will manifest diversity within each developmental period, but the sequence and timing of such periods themselves are viewed to be nearly universal. Much of our late adult lives is considered to be shaped by continuous adaptation to, and accommodation of, decline.

Life-Span Developmental Orientation

In sharp contrast, the life-span developmental orientation (Baltes, 1987; Baltes, Reese, & Lipsitt, 1980) proposes that adaptation and growth of function can occur at any point during the life-span. Later life is not assumed to follow normative or invariant stages of maturation and decline. Instead, the emphasis is on understanding the immense heterogeneity of function, competence, and adaptive potential found in older adults across their later years. Development and qualitative differentiation are viewed as part of a life-long process of gains and losses.

Traditional templates for development in later life are considered unwieldy, given the many anomalies that can result from generational (cohort) differences, accidents of personal history, unique social experience, individual differences in coping, and so on. Moreover, seemingly similar developmental changes may differ across individuals with respect to magnitude, time of onset, or consequences of the change.

The life-span developmental orientation encourages a pluralistic view with respect to potential determinants of individual development. Three general domains of influence have been proposed. The first of these, *normative age-graded* influences, includes a broad mix of biological and environmental factors that are closely related to age. Examples of such influences would include early physical and cognitive maturation processes. They would also include those educational, family, and occupational role involvements that occur at predictable times during the life cycle. The second domain is that of *normative history-graded* influences. These influences are typically associated with a given cohort or generation. They are the defining events or environmental circumstances that might have affected an entire generation and the unfolding of their lives. Such events might include wars, economic depression, or social reform movements such as the struggles for civil rights and women's rights. The third domain involves *nonnormative influences*. Such influences would include those critical life events that are unique to an individual (e.g., an illness, accident, or trauma). They would also include life events that were unique in their timing (e.g., being widowed in early adulthood). Any individual over a lifetime will have experienced a unique history of social involvements, attachments, disappointments, occupational or financial successes and failures, geographic relocations, deaths of loved ones, and so on.

In summary, then, the life-span developmental orientation holds that almost any form of developmental process can occur at any time, for better or worse, in response to a broad mix of internal, external, and historical influences. It would be consistent, then, to expect older adults to experience a diversity of developmental possibilities. In addition, many older adults should be able to remain actively engaged in society until very late in life and to continue to pursue the kinds of goals and relationships they valued in their earlier years (Sterns, 1986). The orientation further implies continued plasticity, the ability to learn and adapt positively to changing life events. Thus, older persons should be able to benefit from the efforts of others to facilitate their well-being and continued development. Providing the support and educational resources to older persons engaged in such efforts would still appear a worthwhile investment (Willis, 1985).

Changing Conceptions of Social Aging

Finally, an analysis of the social meanings of aging helps to place the two previous models of development into some perspective. Neugarten and Neugarten (1986) note that all societies weave age into the process of social organization. We typically classify individuals as being in their childhood, youth, middle, or old age. At times, we make finer distinctions, with reference to their status as an infant, toddler, preteen, young adult, preretiree, and so on.

Within any given culture there has historically been a broad consensus regarding the age boundaries of a group and regarding what constitutes age-appropriate behavior. Chronological age has been used widely as a basis for assigning rights (e.g., to drive, vote, marry, hold public office, retire, or receive social security benefits). It has also been the basis for assigning responsibilities (e.g., age of contractual responsibility, criminal responsibility, military draft eligibility).

Chronological age then has generally served as a useful proxy for more reliable (but more expensive) individualized assessments of maturity, judgment, sense of responsibility, physical or mental status, ability to function competently or contribute productively. In addition, the internalization of a social clock provided for many individuals a point of social comparison, permitting them to evaluate their own progress and accomplishments relative to their age peers. These processes would appear consistent with Levinson's model (discussed above), in which the seasons of a person's life were construed to be shaped by responses to the developmental demands characteristic of a particular chronological period in the life-span.

The Neugartens argue, however, that functional distinctions between age groups have "blurred" in recent decades as society has changed and as more of us are now living significantly longer lives. In particular, with dramatic increases in life expectancy during this century, our conceptions of old age have had to change. Persons over age 65 are now typically active and healthy. Many are capable of remaining in the work force and are motivated to do so. Disabling health declines and dependency are less likely to occur prior to one's early 70s. Many older persons are still members of intact family units, may be preparing to remarry or to reenter an educational or work setting. They do not identify as being old.

Moreover, immense diversity is to be found even among quite old persons. There are of course 75-year-olds who have already retired from occupational and family responsibilities, seeking a more protected life style, perhaps including some form of congregate housing. But, it is not uncommon to find a still vigorous older person who, at the same age, can effectively manage a large corporation or hold the highest political office in the land. The Neugartens have noted that it would now be more useful to think in terms of the "young-old," "middle-old," and "old-old" (the old-old being those who, at whatever their age, have begun to require special health care).

The Neugartens point out that these changing societal trends have introduced greater heterogeneity into society itself, diminishing the social consensus regarding age distinctions and age-appropriate behavior. Internalized social clocks would be expected, therefore, to have less influence as a developmental variable, especially in later life. This interpretation is generally consistent with the life-span developmental orientation, which posits a less universal set of developmental influences in later life and which also proposes that nonnormative developmental factors would begin to exert more influence in old age (Baltes et al., 1980).

NORMATIVE MODELS
OF ADAPTATION AND COPING

Two approaches to adaptation and coping have received considerable attention in the gerontological literature. We turn first to the concept of successful aging, which places adaptation and coping theory in the context of later-life development. Three theoretical approaches to successful aging are particularly heuristic:

Successful Aging

Pfeiffer's Conceptualization of Successful Aging

Pfeiffer (1977) brings a clinical viewpoint to the analysis of successful aging and a concern for psychopathologies likely to result from a failure to adapt successfully to the many negative life changes associated with aging. In the context of anticipated decline in physical, cognitive, and social status, he viewed successful aging in terms of how well one had handled the tasks of adapting to each change in status, minimizing pain and disruption. Adaptation was defined as being able to continue to meet one's physical, psychological, and social needs in the face of recurring loss.

This early model reflects a certain resignation to the sequelae of aging, which include the loss of instrumental competence, relationships, and opportunity to participate in those activities that formerly provided meaning, purpose, stimulation, and reward. Pfeiffer notes a number of important tasks of adaptation. For example, it is important wherever possible to:

- *Replace what has been lost* by finding new social roles or friends to replace those lost after a retirement, bereavement, or relocation.
- *Retrain lost capacities* following an injury or health event, for example, by taking advantage of rehabilitation therapy.
- *Learn to make do with less,* a signal departure from the habitual expectation during earlier life stages that every life change is accompanied by the potential for positive developmental growth.
- *Retain function* by staying aggressively active physically, mentally, and socially; the byword of gerontologists is "use it or lose it."

Pfeiffer notes also that successful adaptation to aging requires certain cognitive and emotional energies. It is important, for example, to take stock continually and to try to achieve some perspective on changes being experienced. It is helpful in this regard to examine issues affecting one's self-concept or identity and to come to some sense of peace with narrowing boundaries of instrumental competence, ability to serve others, diminished physical appearance, and the need to substitute alternatives for formerly rewarding relationships and roles. More broadly, the task is one of finding an acceptable life perspective that balances an appreciation for what went right along the way and a modified view of how one's life can still have purpose and meaning.

Rowe and Kahn's Conceptualization of Successful Aging

Rowe and Kahn (1987) propose a much more aggressive agenda with regard to understanding successful aging. They argue that it is time for researchers to move beyond the strategy of simply mapping the normative (usual) course of age-related decline and loss and focus on the lessons of heterogeneity in aging. Assessments of physiological, psychological, and social function among older persons of the same age exhibit considerable variability, with many individuals showing minimal or no loss. The question is twofold: (1) What portion of "usual" aging effects has been overstated—in that these effects may be in part a function of extrinsic risk factors such as life-style, health behavior, or social integration; and (2) What can we learn from those persons who appear to have aged more successfully than most? Might life-style factors constitute risk factors that could be modified in at-risk populations?

Rowe and Kahn (1987) point to a variety of such factors that appear to modify physiological risks usually associated with aging (e.g., diet, cessation of alcohol consumption or smoking, exercise, and social involvement). They also note a variety of extrinsic influences that appear to minimize the risk of age-related cognitive loss (e.g., education, training to recover lost function, stimulation, improved health, and a socially involved life-style). Examples are also provided of the kinds of factors that have generally been found to enhance social well-being in old age, for example, social support and integration, and feelings of personal control.

The reader will recall that Pfeiffer's (1977) approach to successful aging (discussed above) focused primarily on how best to adapt to the "inevitable" declines and losses associated with aging. That approach reflected a clinical perspective on preventing any psychopathologies associated with failure to adapt to one's constantly changing (declining) status. The point of Rowe and Kahn's approach, however, is that it is important to distinguish between usual and successful aging and then to intensify our investigations of those persons who age more successfully. Such study should identify a wealth of extrinsic factors that influence the trajectory of loss usually associated with aging and suggest intervention strategies by which such factors might be turned to our advantage. Rowe and Kahn's model, then, provides us with a proactive strategy for successful aging that can be enacted in our youth (the earlier the better). We move now to a third model of successful aging, one that emphasizes the human potential to begin aging more successfully *at any point* during the life-span.

Baltes and Baltes's Conceptualization of Successful Aging

Baltes and Baltes (1990) acknowledge the biological changes that accompany aging and implications of these changes for physical, psychological, and social functioning. But, their approach to successful aging focuses on an older person's remaining potential for positive developmental change. Underlying the approach is a growing research base regarding (1) the untapped reserve capacity among older persons, and (2) their potential for continued development and ability to compensate for loss and decline.

For example, the routine activities of daily living (or of most occupations) seldom test the limits of one's full mental capacity. There is now a considerable body of research evidence that older adults are able to continue to learn until quite late in life (see reviews by Willis, 1985, 1987). Within limits, older adults continue to be able to benefit from work-saving technologies, practice and training interventions on cognitive tasks (e.g., Labouvie-Vief, 1985; Schaie & Willis, 1986). Perhaps most exciting is the potential in later life for qualitative development, for example, as in the emergence of wisdom, as older adults successfully integrate a lifetime's experience (e.g., Baltes & Smith, 1990; Labouvie-Vief, 1985; Sternberg, 1990)

Similarly, motor performance and the capacity to perform work in the later years exhibit increasing variability. This reflects age-related physiological changes but also individual differences in activity, motivation, and history of disease (Spirduso & MacRae, 1990). In the absence of disease, aerobic capacity, for example, declines approximately 1% per year after the age of 25; however, if one maintains a constant level of physical activity, that rate of decline may be reduced by one-half (Heath, Hagberg, Ehsani, & Holloszy, 1981). Similar patterns have been found for muscular strength and endurance. Loss of muscle structure and function is lower in older persons who remain active, and exercise has strengthening effects for older adults as well as for younger persons (Spirduso & MacRae, 1990).

Baltes and Baltes suggest a multiple-criteria approach to assessing successful aging, including the individual's status relative to norms on measures of physiological, cognitive, and subjective well-being. They also suggest that criteria include an assessment of the individual's remaining plasticity (the ability to continue to adapt as a changing situation demands).

Behavioral plasticity refers to one's preparedness to adapt. Such preparedness appears to be a matter of one's reserve capacities and strategic process for their utilization. In this context, Baltes and Baltes have proposed a three-part strategy for successful aging (the principle of selective optimization with compensation) that could prove widely useful in older adults' efforts to prolong instrumental functioning and involvement, for example, in their occupation. First, it is important to face the reality that one may no longer be able to do it all—that is, to maintain previous standards of performance across all areas of previous competence or responsibility. The solution is to establish some priorities, to *select* a smaller number of responsibilities or performance domains on which to concentrate all efforts. In doing so, the older person asserts a degree of personal (and strategic) control over the direction of coping efforts. Second, one must find ways to *optimize* performance in the selected domains, such as devoting more time and practice to each of the remaining domains. Third, it will be necessary continually to find ways to *compensate* for declining competence or stamina, making use of technology, other people, and alternative or smarter strategies for accomplishing targeted levels of performance. Baltes and Baltes cite the example of Artur Rubinstein, the pianist, whose strategy for coping with age-related change closely matched the principle of selective optimization with compensation. They report that Rubinstein at some point selected from his extensive repertoire a smaller number of pieces to continue to perform. Then, he increased the amount of practice devoted to these pieces. Finally, he altered his artistic style to give the impression of the great speed that was required for certain movements of a composition. He would noticeably slow his tempo just prior to a faster movement, preparing his audience for a contrast that remained within the somewhat diminished limits of his ability.

Coping with Stressful Life Events

Researchers have also extended broader theories of stress and coping to the aging context. Interesting research has thus focused on identifying stressful life events most relevant to older adults: age-related patterns of coping with stressful life events, daily hassles, and chronic illness; the interrelationships of health, personality, coping style, social support, and so on. A variety of important insights have resulted from this research.

Perhaps the most important theme to emerge (and a theme we return to often in this book) is that continued involvement in caring family relationships entails significant *costs* for older persons, in addition to providing them important benefits. For example, Aldwin and her colleagues (Aldwin, 1990; Colby, Aldwin, Price, & Mishra, 1985) recently developed the Elders Life Stress Inventory to reflect the three groups of stressors most frequently mentioned by their elderly research subjects (their own health and physical functioning, their own personal problems, and the problems being faced by their family members). A large sample of older adults (64% women, mean age = 74) were then asked to rate each life event in terms of its stressfulness. A particularly interesting finding from the study was that, on average, the bad things happening to their loved ones (e.g., a family member's worsening relationship, divorce, deteriorating health, or death) were rated as slightly more stressful than were their own health or personal problems.

Another central theme concerns the relative uncontrollability of many of the stressors characteristic of old age and how that might influence the nature of coping among older persons. In later life, accumulating stressors (e.g., chronic illness, diminished physiological functioning, loss of loved ones, financial decline) are viewed as less changeable. It seems reasonable, therefore, that older persons also appear less likely than younger persons to adopt an active, problem-solving approach to coping (Brandtstadter & Renner, 1990; Felton, 1990; Folkman, Lazarus, Pimley, & Novacek, 1987). Rather, they are likely to adopt an accommodative, emotion-focused coping strategy, recognizing and accepting the limitations of the new situation, reappraising the stressor as less traumatic than previously feared, finding a positive side to the situation, trying not to remain upset, and so on (Brandtstadter & Renner, 1990; Felton, 1990; Folkman et al., 1987).

This tendency to a more accommodative coping strategy may be difficult to reconcile with the various models of successful aging discussed above. A timely adoption of an accommodative strategy and the implications for minimizing undue psychological distress associated with decline would be consistent with Pfeiffer's (1977) model. Yet, premature adoption would seem to be the whole point of both the approaches of Rowe and Kahn (1987) and Baltes and Baltes (1990).

But, in old age the concept of active compensatory strategies may be more broadly construed. There comes a time (e.g., in case of chronic illness or disability) when direct coping action against the stressor becomes infeasible. At such a time, older persons are likely to refocus coping efforts to alternative coping resources. For most, the predominant such resource will involve one's family and social relationships (e.g., Felton, 1990). Attention will thus need to focus on assessing current family and social networks and their support potential. Where that support potential is appraised as insufficient for one's changing needs, it will become necessary to think about how to construct or access new social networks, and how to ensure the stability, supportive capacity, and good will of such networks over the long term. This process is problematic. It is influenced by the characteristics of the illness or situation, the characteristics of the potentially supportive network, and the characteristics of the older person requiring assistance. These issues have received considerable research attention, to which we now turn.

CHAPTER 3

The Problematic Nature of Supportive Relationships in Old Age

We explored in Chapters 1 and 2 how personal relationships facilitate support and adaptation among older adults. This growing body of evidence regarding the positive effects of family and social support has greatly influenced health care and social service practitioners. One example of this is the increasing incorporation of assessments of family relationships into the process of hospital discharge planning for elderly patients. This process involves analyses of the patient's continuing needs and ability to cope in the environment to which the individual must return. In planning a case-management strategy, therefore, it is typical to assess the patient's social resources along with medical and functional status (Kane & Kane, 1981).

Unfortunately, the relationships on which support depends can often be problematic, undermining the ability of family, friends, and more formal networks to serve in this role. Such concerns may be compounded among older persons, whose demands on their networks may also be changing in ways that increasingly reflect chronic distress and diminished resources for social exchange.

If the continuity and stability of important support relationships can not be taken for granted, a variety of consequences could follow, with certain classes of older persons being at greater risk. Such consequences often are counterintuitive, reflect subtle social process, and require that we reexamine our theoretical assumptions about helping relationships. Research, clinical examples, and a number of theoretical papers regarding such concerns in helping relationships are now beginning to appear. In this chapter, we discuss many examples as they reflect the broader interpersonal context, and in Chapter 4, we focus on concerns specific to the family.

We introduce in this chapter four general themes regarding the problematic nature of supportive relationships in old age. First, among these is the likelihood of *relational loss;* the frequency of deaths among friends and relatives increases in later years. Relational loss thus tends to cluster in old age, requiring extraordinary coping efforts at a time when the major players in one's support network are being lost. The next two themes involve age-related barriers to maintaining personal relationships and to developing new ones when necessary. Such barriers may reflect such *personal vulnerabilities* as the deterioration of physical health, changing psychological status (loneliness, depression, isolation, etc.), or shifting needs and priorities. They may also reflect *environmental barriers* such as diminished economic status, mobility or access, and the stereotypic attitudes of society toward the aged. Finally, we explore the potential for *stress and conflict* within existing personal and family relationships of the elderly.

CONVOYS OF SOCIAL SUPPORT

It is important to remember that a person's needs, relationships, and social networks tend to evolve and change across a lifetime. At different points in our lives, our networks will vary in size, complexity, stability, and function (Antonucci, 1985). Age-normative events such as marriage, having children and grandchildren, entering the workplace, and becoming involved in civic life provide new connections and opportunities for social integration. But, many of the events characteristic of later life, such as diminished health and mobility, reduced income, retirement from the workplace, or the death of friends and family can disrupt the form, function, and effectiveness of our networks.

Kahn and Antonucci (1980) have used the term "convoys of social support" to denote the dynamic nature and patterning of an individual's social relationships across the life course. Antonucci (1985) summarized much of the literature on support networks across the lifespan, providing a number of useful, empirical generalizations that are discussed below.

Network size (number of potentially supportive family members or friends) seems not to change significantly with age, although the amount of support exchanged may decrease somewhat. However, women tend to have larger, more diverse networks than do men. Similarly, women list more persons among their networks who serve as a trusted confidant. This reflects in part the greater tendency of women to develop support relationships with friends, as well as family. It also appears to reflect more effective social skills on the part of wom en. A broader, more intimate and flexible network should provide a buffer against the loss of key family members in later years and should make it more likely that the appropriate form of support would be available and sufficient when needed (Hobfoll, 1988).

Among older persons, relationships with friends increase in importance relative to relationships with kin. But, the instrumental support relationships of frail, declining elderly persons appear to follow fairly predictable patterns. Primary care typically falls first to a spouse (often of similar age and degree of frailty), then to children and immediate relatives, and then increasingly involves more formal health care and housing entities.

Persons of higher economic status and education tend to have larger, less dense networks. Members of their networks are therefore less likely to know or be connected to one another, but they are likely to represent a broader range of available support resources.

Finally, the relationships summarized above remain to be systematically assessed with respect to their stability across ethnic groups. For example, research is beginning to suggest that the nature and meaning of stressful life events (e.g., bereavement) can vary across cultures, that it is often difficult to know how another person feels in their aftermath, and that both personal and more formal support systems may need to reexamine their assumptions for providing support across ethnic lines (Lopata, 1988; Rosenblatt, 1988). Similarly, our assumptions regarding the "normative" nature and functioning of support systems are probably too limited. For example, African-Americans, compared to whites, are more likely to incorporate into their support networks an extended mix of *fictive kin* or *para-kin* (e.g., friends, and members of their church and community) who provide a network of considerably greater depth and flexibility (George, 1988; Johnson & Barer, 1990; Sussman, 1985). In contrast, in more patriarchal cultures such as India, Korea, or Turkey, a widow will traditionally be economically dependent, and will likely enter her son's or her late husband's family household (Lopata, 1987).

RELATIONAL LOSS

Our relationships across the life-span provide important elements of our well-being. They reflect the manner in which societies organize themselves to maintain the social order as well as the ability of individuals to participate and contribute effectively. Theory-driven research on social support and applied research by gerontologists suggests that it generally goes well. In later life, however, there are recurring demands on the individual to accommodate change in the structure and composition of relational networks, to manage transition, and to deal with relational loss through death. As substantial portions of our social networks will be comprised of persons with whom we share an intense emotional attachment, relational loss will at times be traumatic (Bowlby, 1969, 1973, 1980; Weiss, 1988). The import of such issues can easily be seen, for example, in the case of bereavement.

The consequences of bereavement have been studied most extensively with respect to widowhood, which occurs most frequently in later life. More than 50% of American women and 12% of men aged 65 or older have become widowed (U.S. Bureau of the Census, 1984a). Considerable clinical research has now focused on the symptomatology and course of bereavement (e.g., Gallagher-Thompson, Futterman, Farberow, Thompson, & Peterson, 1993; Lund, Caserta, & Dimond, 1993; Stroebe & Stroebe, 1987, 1993). In such studies, bereavement reactions are commonly found to involve a broad array of emotional, cognitive, and behavioral disturbances and an increased risk for deteriorating physical health and mortality (Stroebe & Stroebe, 1987; Stroebe, Stroebe, & Hansson, 1993). Of particular interest, however, the timing and incidence of conjugal bereavement are unequally distributed across subsets of the population. As Table 3.1 illustrates, for example, women and ethnic minorities are widowed earlier.

AGE-RELATED BARRIERS TO DEVELOPING AND MAINTAINING RELATIONSHIPS: BROADER THEMATIC ISSUES

The notion of convoys of support described above implies that our relationships across a lifetime will involve considerable turnover and the need to manage difficult transitions. We have suggested that many persons will do that well, but some persons and classes of persons are likely to be at increased risk for poor outcome.

TABLE 3.1. Percentage of Widowed Persons Aged 55 and Over by Race and Sex (1982)

Age	White males (%)	White females (%)	Black males (%)	Black females (%)
55–64	3.1	16.4	7.8	26.0
65–74	6.9	37.4	15.7	47.3
75 +	20.6	67.6	34.0	77.9

Source: U.S. Bureau of the Census. (1984b). *Marital Status and Living Arrangements: Current Population Reports, March 1982.* Washington, DC: U.S. Government Printing Office.

Role Contraction across the Life Course

An additional body of theory from the sociology of aging suggests even more systematic concerns regarding our access in later life to satisfying and helpful relationships. Sociologist Irving Rosow (1985) proposed that later life is a time in which our social roles systematically contract in ways that exclude older persons from meaningful social interaction. In early and middle adulthood, people typically assume a wide variety of important, functional roles that have a well defined (institutionalized) status. For these roles (such as spouse, parent, employee, military reservist, or school board member), there are typically clear expectations regarding the nature and scope of one's responsibilities and normative standards for performance. Such roles provide tangible, but also intangible, rewards (e.g., self-esteem, a sense of structure, predictability, and belonging).

Rosow argues that in later life people become less involved in these institutionalized roles, tending rather to enter (or be relegated to) roles whose functions are mostly token or symbolic and that make fewer meaningful demands for competence or responsibility. Thus, a greater proportion of our time is spent in such roles as parent of adult children, grandparent, ex-spouse, widow, retired worker, and so forth.

A number of important implications might be drawn regarding this phenomenon. In a sense, the role behavior and performance of older adults could become less "socially consequential." Their inclusion and interaction in the social group might become dependent more on protocol, tradition, and good will rather than on their potential to contribute or exercise influence in any meaningful way. There should be fewer serious normative expectations from the group regarding their participation or contributions; their social status, power, and available resources for social exchange within the group should also be reduced.

Diminishing Peer Networks

We noted earlier in the book (see Chapter 1), that in later life the importance of companionship and social support from age-peers increases and that of kin decreases. However, the risk in very old age involves the aging of the support network itself and the loss of many of these old friends. Anthropologist Barbara Myerhoff (1978) addressed this concern in a compelling account of an elderly Jewish community in Venice, California. The men and women she studied were European emigres, approximately 80 years of age. Their children and grandchildren had completely assimilated into the American culture—a matter of immense pride among the community. An inevitable cost in the process, however, was that their children had also distanced themselves from the orthodox religion and culture, and from the language in which the elders felt most comfortable. Thus, peer relationships became of utmost importance as these elderly persons strove to remain independent, to preserve their ways and their dignity. They would gather daily at the community center to socialize and to participate in the culture. They enjoyed many of the benefits of personal and community relationships (companionship, stimulation, emotional and instrumental support, and at times intense political confrontation). They were proud when the level of their contributions to others was greater than benefits they derived. Of greatest importance, however, they shared a sense of cohort. This tiny, rather isolated community provided a cherished sense of belonging, of ties to their cultural and religious history. It also provided a relatively safe haven from which to deal with the sometimes threatening, outside world.

Yet, this tightly bounded support network was itself aging and members were dying. Much of its attention, therefore, was necessarily devoted to demands for adaptation and survival on the part of not only individuals, but the group itself. The focus and functions of the center, and cultural and religious traditions long cherished were subtly altered to serve the remaining members and the newly precarious position of the group. Goals and scope of activities were continually redrawn inward to reflect the more realistic circumstances of a frail, elderly membership. At the level of the group, then, their coping efforts and stratagems seemed much like Pfeiffer's (1977) suggestions to aging individuals (i.e., replace lost resources with new, work vigorously to retain abilities as long possible, retrain lost abilities where possible, and find ways, with dignity and meaning, to learn to do with less).

We believe that Meyerhoff's account provides a model for understanding the circumstances of many elderly in today's society. Long-standing personal associations tend to age and change in function and utility via such processes as their members near the end of their lives. The implication is that the practical value of these relationships will diminish for the last remaining members at the time of their greatest need.

Strained Relationships in Later Life

Researchers have also become interested in the strains inherent in personal relationships in later life. Such strains can reflect the nature of friendship itself but also the characteristics of the individuals involved.

Rook (1989) recently summarized the research regarding factors with the particular potential to undermine friendships in later life. The following themes follow closely her analysis: Unlike family relationships, friendships are voluntary. They lack the symbolic or contractual commitments that might assist in surviving troubled or conflicted times. Friendships also are usually a source of both rewards and costs, positive, but also troublesome interactions. For example, when friends (like family) become involved in providing social support, well-meaning efforts may be accompanied by invasions of privacy, feelings of frustration and anger, broken promises, unwanted advice or assistance (Rook, 1984; Stephens, Kinney, Ritchie, & Norris, 1987). When negative exchanges do occur, the consequences can outweigh any benefits derived from the relationship (Rook, 1984).

Non-kin friendships become especially important sources of companionship and comfort in later life. However, the accumulation of relational loss that will have occurred to older persons may render them particularly sensitive to strains in current relationships.

In old age, it is more likely that instrumental support will be provided by kin, and companionship by friends. However, in the absence of kin, older persons may need to call upon friends for instrumental support. Such violations of normative expectations might be expected to create strain and feelings of resentment within the friendship (Rook, 1987).

Dramatic life or health events (e.g., illness or a bereavement) may irreversibly diminish one's physical, social, or economic resources in later life. Such occurrences to one member of a friendship limit the potential for a reciprocally rewarding relationship. Disruptive strains such as these could therefore result in diminished contact between friends in the short term, and in the longer run, they could lead to a reduction of personal investment in or termination of the relationship. In this connection, Connidis and Davies (1992) found evidence that among older adults aged 65–92 years, increasing age was associated with a reduced probability of having a friend who provides companionship or serves as a confidant. Their interpretation of this pattern was that it reflected in part a declining pool of available friends, increased strains on friendships in later life, and a return to reliance on family for these intimate needs.

Finally, the experience of chronic stress among older people may actually function to produce social isolation rather than an automatic search for intimate ties and social support. For example, Krause (1991) found evidence that among persons with an average age of 66 years, financial strain and fear of neighborhood crime were significantly related to an increased distrust of other people, and to feelings that one had no one to call on or count on in times of trouble. A path analysis of the data also showed that financial strain and fear of crime were related directly to social isolation, but they were also indirectly related to social isolation through their influence on distrust. Krause concluded that, ironically, chronic stress may actually erode the social resources that could assist the individual to cope with the stress.

Interpersonal Betrayals in Later-Life Relationships

The preceding analyses suggest primarily structural concerns and the limitations of well-meaning persons in relationships. The analyses reflect systemic problems with the continued competence and endurance of the individuals involved that might be expected to occur in later life. However, we have also studied in elderly adults the kinds of relational strain that reflect the darker side of personal relationships (Hansson, Jones, & Fletcher, 1990). As is the case with relationships involving younger persons, older people (by disposition or circumstance) often become involved in conflict, deception, or violations of trust. The consequences of such eruptions in an older person's relationships can be especially threatening, given an increasing dependency on family and social networks for instrumental support.

Our research in this area focused on the manner and degree to which older adults experience interpersonal betrayal in their relationships. We asked 60 people (average age = 68 years) to describe an incident from their lives that they considered to be their own most significant act of betrayal and also to describe an incident in which they felt they had been betrayed. Upon completing their narrative, they responded to questions about the relationships involved, motivations, and consequences.

Analyses of the incidents reported suggested a number of patterns. It was clear that issues of interpersonal trust were meaningful to this population; 48 of the 60 were able to describe an incident of betrayal (although approximately half of these were from their earlier years). Respondents reported having betrayed 14% of the people in their networks and having been betrayed by nearly 20%. Their betrayals of others most often involved either extramarital affairs (20.5%) or telling lies (20.5%). Another 10.3% involved broken promises, and 7.7% involved betrayals of a confidence. Betrayals of the respondent by others most frequently involved being cheated out of money (15%), extramarital affairs (12.5%), being lied to (12.5%), and betrayals of a confidence (12.5%).

Members of immediate family (potentially important members of one's support network in old age) were most often the victim of respondent's incidents of betrayal. They were also the most frequent source of betrayal. In addition, nearly two-thirds of the respondents indicated that their victims had known about the betrayal, undermining the support potential of their family support system. For example, those who reported having betrayed a greater proportion of their support network also indicated that they had been the victim of betrayal more frequently, and they reported more disagreements in the network.

Changing Social Worlds: Modernization

In a rapidly changing society, every generation of the very old will eventually face a gap between the social world into which they were socialized and the world in which they must cope in old age. Modernity theorists and researchers have widely documented many of the broader issues in this respect (cf. Finley, 1982). In practical terms, breakthroughs in health technology during the last half-century have increased longevity, and therefore the burden of social security and health care costs on society. Advances in industrial technologies have resulted in a more rapidly changing economic environment, fostering occupational obsolescence and lower status among older adults. The urbanization of society and movement away from an agrarian base encouraged a migration of family members (especially younger members) to urban industrial centers, separating parents physically from the families of their children.

These issues also suggest a number of concerns that relate more directly to the support functions of older persons' relational networks. For instance, their children's attention will generally be focused elsewhere (on their own lives, children, and careers); society's professional helpers and gatekeepers (health practitioners, social service personnel, etc.) will be of a younger generation, with new perspectives, priorities, and methods; and a good portion of one's old friends will have died or moved away. Such age-related factors might be expected to isolate many older persons in need from the community's support resources.

In this connection, Lopata (1988) described an important source of social isolation from her studies of elderly urban widows. She points out older adults in the United States often were raised in small, tightly woven communities where everyone was widely known and naturally occurring support systems were highly attentive to one's needs. However, societal structure changed with increased industrial modernization, urbanization, and mobility of families. As a consequence, it can no longer be taken for granted that all persons in need (especially those of low status or those without kin) will be noticed, much less helped. Today's more loosely woven communities are less likely to reach out to all of their members in need. Therefore, the elderly must take the initiative in establishing and maintaining the kinds of friendships and social networks that can be called on when needed. Lopata notes that these kinds of efforts, required in a voluntaristic society, will be especially difficult for older women who may not have been encouraged in their youth to explore aggressively and to initiate new relationships outside of the home and family.

Stereotyped Perceptions and Attitudes Regarding Older Adults

Older adults are a highly diverse population in terms of their psychological, physical health, and socioeconomic status. Much age-related change in these domains appears to be multidetermined, and individual vulnerability differs across individuals and classes of individuals, resulting in increased heterogeneity in the later years. Some older persons do experience early decrements in cognitive or physical functioning, but a large number retain and even improve in status in certain functions until very late in life. In addition, many of the declines previously attributed to the normal aging process appear to result from pathological conditions that are modifiable, or that might have been deferred or prevented (cf. Rowe & Kahn, 1987). Rowe and Kahn note, for example, a variety of factors that predict more successful aging with respect to cognitive, emotional, and health stability (e.g., exercise, diet, health habits, access to health care, amount of stimulation, social support, and personal control). Such variables of course are unevenly distributed, placing socially isolated individuals or persons of lower socioeconomic status, for example, at greater risk.

In spite of this diversity, however, the elderly are commonly subject to stereotyped perceptions. Of particular concern, age-related stereotypes may place elderly individuals at considerable risk because they lead to an unexamined response to changes in the older person's health or psychological status. That is, the older adult, family members and even health-care professionals may assume, erroneously, that new symptoms are simply the natural and irreversible consequences of aging. Older adults have been found not to have sought professional evaluation of new symptoms for exactly this reason (Nuttbrock & Kosberg, 1980), and professionals have conducted less rigorous clinical assessments of patients where the presenting symptoms could be considered symptomatic of aging (Butler, 1975). Similarly, well-meaning family members may provide too comprehensive a level of support, precluding the older parent's own efforts to cope with a new health status, encouraging a premature sense of dependency (Kahn, 1975) and undermining the older person's sense of autonomy (Rowe & Kahn, 1987). Recent research examples of such disruptive influences in health care and support will be presented later in this chapter.

Age-related stereotypes also have consequences for society at large. As we noted in Chapter 2, societies historically have used age as an element of social organization. A consensus emerges, is institutionalized, and passed down the generations regarding the roles, norms, and behaviors that are to be associated with a given age.

As we have seen, however, these seemingly clear historical patterns have begun to blur as society becomes more complex. As members of modern society begin to live longer, earlier assumptions about age-appropriate phases of life become less useful. Many individuals now are relatively healthy and competent to remain in the work force and other instrumental family and societal roles well beyond their 60s and 70s.

Neugarten and Neugarten (1986) argue that our emergence as a more complex society requires that we consider individuals and their varying needs rather than use age as a proxy for judgments of competence. They suggest further that we must reexamine those age-assumptions by which society assigns rights, protections, and access to resources but which may also become a source of age discrimination. It is noteworthy, however, that ageist stereotypes and their consequences persist. In 1986, for example, over 26,000 age discrimination in employment cases were filed in the United States. This is approximately twice the number of cases filed in 1980. Moreover, in 1986, one in four cases filed by the Equal Employment Opportunity Commission concerned age discrimination in employment (Freedberg, 1987).

Stereotyping in Health Care Contexts

Age-related stereotypes can have especially important consequences when they find their way into health care contexts, where frail elderly are more dependent on others to help them to understand and cope with stressful circumstances. Research on the quality and effectiveness of such relationships often points to the vulnerability of older adults when they are unable to assert their needs and rights within the health care system.

The difficulties encountered by older persons in health care settings reflect in part a lack of attention on the part of health professionals and institutions and a continuing disinterest in older patients. As early as 1975, Robert Butler (the founding director of the National Institute of Aging) described such attitudes among physicians with respect to older patients. He attributed such attitudes to a number of potential factors. For example, older patients are likely to have sensory problems and difficulty in communicating their symptoms. They may also have different values or health beliefs from their physicians, who may be from a different generation and a different socioeconomic class. It is also relevant that older patients may be viewed as less convenient, requiring more of the physician's time, emergency visits, more frequent hospitalizations, and fee billings subject to oversight (and caps) by government agencies.

Compounding the problem are the ways in which the illness experience of older adults differs from younger persons. In old age, there is added concern for chronic health conditions and disabilities (e.g., arthritis, heart disease, hypertension, hearing impairment, or diabetes). Such conditions must be managed carefully to maximize continuing functional ability, and they increase an older adult's vulnerability to acute illness or trauma (Rowe, 1985). Moreover, illness in old age is more likely to result from a combination of interacting physiological factors, rather than from an infection or the deterioration of a single system. In addition, the symptoms of many diseases in elderly persons are often different from those seen in younger persons. For example, presenting symptoms of myocardial infarction in older persons are less likely to involve discernible chest pain, but rather confusion, disorientation, and more general weakness (Rowe, 1985). Thus, pathological conditions are often less specific, harder to diagnose and to treat.

Adding to this complexity are the intensifying interrelationships (with age) among physical, psychological, and social functioning (Cohen, 1990; Gatz & Smyer, 1992). Diminished health and sensory status can have an impact on intellectual functioning, social competence, and mobility (Schaie, 1981). In addition, life events characteristic of later life, for example, bereavement, disability, or retirement can result in a diminished sense of control, depression, altered health behavior, modulation of immune and endocrine systems, and increased risk of physical morbidity (Kemp, 1985; Laudenslager, 1988; Stroebe & Stroebe, 1987).

Dealing with the health care needs of older persons is thus highly complex. It requires a genuine sensitivity and interest in their needs, coordinated, multidisciplinary assessments of their physical, cognitive, and social functioning, and goals for case management and rehabilitation that are realistic (Kemp, 1985). It is therefore understandable that researchers and clinicians continue to document regrettable and often ironic failures of the system. We present a few examples below as illustration.

Health care professionals may also systematically underestimate an older patient's competence or potential for rehabilitation. In this connection, Barta Kvitek, Shaver, Blood, and Shepard (1986) studied physical therapists in 14 hospitals and rehabilitation facilities. The therapists were asked to read a detailed patient description, including information on the patient's disabling injury, medical response thus far, and pertinent psychological and social factors (the patient was described as either 28 or 78 years of age; otherwise patient descriptions were identical). They were then asked to recommend rehabilitation goals for the patient with respect to ability to ambulate and perform the activities of daily living, recommended frequency and rigor of therapy, and return to home and independent living. Those therapists who thought they were evaluating an older patient recommended significantly less aggressive rehabilitation goals. Of particular interest, however, among therapists who evaluated the older patient, those who exhibited a less positive attitude toward aging in general, recommended less aggressive goals.

A related example of unintentional influences on medical judgments was provided by Morgan (1985). This study involved the judgments of nursing staff in British nursing homes regarding mental confusion among their elderly residents. Mental confusion is often multidetermined in older persons with potential causes including organic disorder, but also malnutrition, mismedication, or interacting medications, substance abuse, depression, lack of mobility or stimulation, and so forth (American Psychiatric Association, 1987). Nevertheless, judgments on the part of nursing staff regarding a patient's mental competence tend to influence that patient's care and management in basic ways. A problem confirmed in Morgan's study, however, is that judgments of confusion may be premature. In this case (controlling statistically for actual level of objectively assessed confusion), patients with more limited ability to perform the physical activities of daily living (ADL) were also judged to experience increased problems with communication, which in turn predicted nurses' ratings of increased mental confusion.

Conclusions regarding irreversible cognitive decline, inappropriately based on information regarding very different limitations are a matter of great concern for older adults. But, stereotypic perceptions of elderly nursing home residents and their needs may also be fostered by the nursing home culture itself. Residents will have moved into highly standardized living spaces with little room for personal possessions (symbolic links to one's personal history; Kamptner, 1989). Moreover, institutional pressures to manage the delivery of services to residents in a manner that minimizes cost and disruption to routine are unlikely to encourage highly individualized care. It is interesting, therefore, that if a patient's uniqueness and life history are shared with nursing staff, and the sense of anonymity lifted, perceptions can change. Pietrukowicz and Johnson (1991) found that if nurses' aides were able to read a brief description of a patient's life history (major life events and milestones, interests, beliefs, habits, etc.), they rated the patient as more instrumentally competent, independent, and socially adaptable. Such positive perceptions, like negative stereotypes, would be expected to influence staff attitudes and treatment of the patient.

Strained Relationships in Health Care Settings

Relationships with health professionals can also become strained when conflicts arise regarding treatment alternatives or the older patient's competence and autonomy in decision making. At such times, negotiations may involve the older patient, a professional charged with case management, and other interested parties, such as family members. For example, approximately 20% of the time a relative or friend accompanies the older patient to the appointment with a physician (Adelman, Greene, & Charon, 1987). The third person is typically present in the role of supportive advocate, but there is occasionally a hidden agenda. This individual may wish to be involved in any decision regarding treatment, housing, or institutionalization options. However, the presence of the third party may also inhibit the functional relationship between patient and health practitioner by making it more difficult to disclose symptoms, discuss personal feelings or embarrassing, age- or illness-related problems. Such interference could undermine the development of trust in the medical interaction, with subsequent implications for patient cooperation and adherence to prescribed treatment. It would be helpful at times like this if the older patient could establish some ground rules for the interaction. Too frequently, however, the older person is highly dependent upon both the informal and formal support systems and will be unable to assert much control. It is consistent that older patients report being less likely to change doctors following an upsetting experience during a medical visit (Hansson, Remondet, Obrochta, & Bell, 1988).

As constrained as interpersonal involvement with health practitioners can be, the older persons discussed above at least had access to health care settings. A large number of the elderly do not have such formal relationships, and to fill the gap, the American health care system provides many kinds of community outreach programs. These programs can be effective in early detection, and periodic monitoring of health conditions among the elderly (Rubenstein, Josephson, Nichol-Seamons, & Robbins, 1986). However, in such programs, available resources seldom permit a thorough and active search for all persons in need. They are typically housed in a local community or nutrition center to which one must travel on a voluntary basis. Some elderly persons will simply not hear about the available services, some will not identify as "old" or "poor," and thus feel uncomfortable receiving such services. Some will be too frail. In this connection, a national conference on the special needs of older women in America, expressed as a priority concern the situation of older women, who in very late life may be widowed, have limited economic resources, and live in social isolation (National Institue on Aging, 1978).

Additional conflicts are likely to arise as older adults become more frail and require some protection and assistance in living. In very old age, dependency and need for care are likely to be progressive. As such, the demands on caregivers, health practitioners, or residential staff become more intense, as do the pressures to become more directly involved in decision making for the older person. Over 70% of the adult children of such elderly persons acknowledge that at some point in this process they intend to become involved in their parents' decision making (Hansson, Nelson, et al., 1990). The primary triggers for such involvement are typically health-related ones, but the issue can also become salient in the event of a disruption to the older person's support system (e.g., with the death of a spouse–caregiver, or when housing or neighborhood conditions become too dangerous for the older family member to negotiate safely).

However, there is often disagreement between adult children and the older parent regarding the parent's continuing competence to live independently. Independence may be fiercely defended, as the last symbolic vestige of not being old, or the older person simply may not have noticed important decrements in performance (e.g., in driving; Sterns, Barrett, & Alexander, 1985). Families must therefore consider the relative importance of safety and health care designed to prolong life versus the older parent's needs and desires for independence. Such issues are difficult and often violate, for the first time, established roles and democratic family traditions for decision making. Health practitioners, such as gerontological nurses, have now begun to search for ways to assist families in solving such problems in a manner that is sensitive to the wide range of practical and ethical issues involved (e.g., Hogstel & Gaul, 1991).

Similar concerns also arise after an older person has entered congregate housing or a nursing home. At this point, it is more clear that the individual has entered a continuum of care that will eventually involve a sequence of moves, from relative independence to living circumstances that more directly reflect one's medical needs. Entry into a continuum-of-care residential setting typically assumes that at some point there will be increased frailty and movement along the continuum. The more frail the older person at the time, the more involved and responsible the nursing and residential staff are going to be in decisions about the process. Yet, for many older adults, having to move to a higher-level care facility is frightening and repulsive (involving loss of privacy, freedom, and last remaining personal possessions); it is to be delayed at all costs (Morgan, 1982). In this connection, Morgan notes a variety of strategies that residents often use, to include disguising new health problems, minimizing their consequences by enlisting additional forms of social or instrumental support, or seeking outside help to override the plans of nursing or administrative staff. Professional staff are thus faced with their responsibility to move the resident to a more intense nursing area of the facility in order to extend life, whereas the patient views the transfer as "social death" (Morgan, 1982, p. 48).

The previous section dealt with those structural aspects of an older person's life circumstances that could directly undermine important decision making. However, a variety of subtle strains on personal relationships with coresidents or with health care workers in home or residential settings have also been found to influence the older patient's care and level of well-being. For example, the United States currently devotes a considerable portion of publicly assisted housing to the elderly. An underlying assumption is that living with same-age peers will foster social interaction, buffer against loneliness, and provide additional social support networks. Unfortunately, such goals are not always realized. In fact, residents of senior housing continue to receive most of their social support from family members (Stephens & Bernstein, 1984). This reflects in part the security of older, more predictable relationships and the tendency of friendships not to form quickly.

Moreover, those older residents most in need of support, that is, those with more advanced health conditions or impairments often seem the least likely to be involved in relationships where they might receive it (Stephens & Bernstein, 1984). The social isolation of these frailer residents reflects feelings and choices on their own part, but also on the part of younger, healthier residents (Sheehan, 1986). That is, older and frailer residents report feeling unable to keep up socially with younger counterparts and a reluctance to ask for help. In addition, they expect to be discriminated against by younger residents on the basis of their health status, and they see little value in trying to replace long-standing relationships of known quality with short-term relationships. Younger residents, on the other hand, take their remaining moments of independence very seriously and seem reluctant to become overly involved with frail residents. This would appear to reflect an emotional distancing from reminders of what's to come, but it also reflects a realistic assessment of their own limited coping resources and the likelihood that a support relationship with frailer residents would not be reciprocal (Sheehan, 1986). Such influences then raise barriers to the formation of friendship and support relationships between residents in congregate senior housing, isolating especially those who are in greatest need. It should therefore be a goal in such environments to find ways to reduce the costs of forming supportive, informal relationships.

Relationships with Health Care Workers

Finally, personal relationships that develop between older patients and health care workers are also extremely important, in that they can facilitate communication, trust, and case management. For example, in a study of home health aides and personal care attendants, Eustis and Fischer (1991) found that caregiving services tended to cross formal contractual guidelines. That is, such persons often felt like, and were regarded more like, a friend; they would, for example provide extra services and companionship. Three quarters of the aides surveyed reported serving as a trusted confidant in matters of emotional or personal distress.

The development of a genuine personal relationship under such circumstances, however, can be undermined by subtle social process. In the Eustis and Fischer study, aides usually recognized that their relationship with the physically dependent patient was nonreciprocal. In addition, they often expressed concern that it was hard to maintain clear boundaries between professional responsibilities and personal relationships. To some aides the job was a simply a job, and demands for more personal relationships could become exploitive. In contrast, for the client, it sometimes became difficult to monitor and enforce job performance standards with a friend.

Similar issues arise between residents of nursing homes and the nursing assistants with whom they have close personal contact. Recent reports (e.g., Institute of Medicine, 1986) have emphasized the importance of warm, respectful relationships between nursing home personnel and residents in the latter's adjustment and well-being. Relationships with staff would seem especially critical, given the common finding that many residents are unwilling or unable to form relationships with other residents. For example, Retsinas and Garrity (1985) found about 35% of nursing home residents to have no friends in the home. A study by Wells and Macdonald (1981) found over 50% of residents who could not name someone with whom they were close. Bitzan and Kruzich (1990) in a study of 54 nursing homes found only about 40% of residents who felt close to a fellow resident. In this study, males, persons with lower mental status, and those who experienced greater hearing or ambulation disabilities were less likely to feel close to someone in the home.

It is therefore clear that peer relationships in nursing homes tend not to be strong, or to systematically provide needed companionship or social support. Such needs might thus be expected to be met by staff or administration. Yet, relationships with nursing home staff can also be problematic. For example, residents and nursing assistants are often dissimilar in age, race, religion, and marital status (Heiselman & Noelker, 1991). Heiselman and Noelker surveyed residents and nursing assistants about these issues. Nursing assistants generally welcomed a close personal relationship with their clients; over 90% expected to be like family. It is interesting, however, that these expectations were shared only by about one-half of the residents. The other half felt the need for some social distance from staff and wanted service, not a personal relationship from staff. In this connection, many of the nursing assistants reporting experiencing disrespect and social distancing on the part of residents and their families. In fact, 45% had been accused by residents and their families of providing inadequate care or of stealing from the resident.

Such a difficult social climate in the workplace would understandably be stressful for nursing home staff. In combination with the heavy physical demands of the job, and the low wages and low status often associated with nursing home employment, such conditions could undermine quality of care. It should not be surprising then, that a recent study of 577 nurses and nursing aides in such facilities found considerable evidence of elder patient abuse (Pillemer & Moore, 1989). Thirty-six percent of respondents in this study had witnessed at least one case of physical abuse in the previous year (e.g., excessive restraint, pushing, hitting a patient), and 81% had witnessed at least one incident involving psychological abuse (e.g., yelling, insulting, swearing at a patient, or threatening to deny food or privileges). Of particular interest in the present context, self-reported abuse by respondents was not significantly related to the structural characteristics of the nursing homes involved (e.g., smaller size, lower rates, for-profit) or to characteristics of the employee usually thought to affect general quality of care (e.g., younger, less educated, or less experienced). Instead, the likelihood of abuse was significantly related to reports of interpersonal conflict with patients, feelings of job burnout, frequent thoughts of quitting, a stressful personal life off the job, and to beliefs that older patients were like children — and often in need of discipline (Pillemer & Moore, 1989).

In this chapter we have introduced a number of thematic, problematic influences on the personal and support relationships of older adults, and their implications within broader social contexts. In the next chapter, we examine these issues within the family systems of elderly persons, with specific emphasis on the obstacles they raise for social support and caregiving. In this context, also, we will explore related support issues for the bereaved.

Obstacles to Family Support and Caregiving in Later Years

I t is the premise of this book that relationships serve many critical functions for older adults. Evidence abounds regarding the spirit in which people working with family, or through various forms of voluntary association, support one another in time of greatest need. We saw in Chapter 3, however, how relationships in the broader community may sometimes fail to serve these functions adequately. In the present chapter, we extend that analysis to examine obstacles to family support and caregiving in later life. The reader will note in the process that such obstacles reflect structural limitations inherent to most forms of social organization but also the increased likelihood in times of stress that even family relationships may take on a toxic element.

FAMILY SUPPORT ISSUES IN LATER LIFE

As we have seen, most older adults are not socially isolated. Families continue to be heavily involved in providing social and caregiver support, although the nature of such relationships is typically one of exchange, with elders continuing to contribute their share long after their children have grown and established their own families (Brody, 1985; Cantor, 1991; Kingson, et al., 1986; Mitchell & Register, 1984; Stone, Cafferata, & Sangl, 1987).

It has also become clear, however, that in old age the nature of dependency upon support networks may change dramatically, reflecting the onset of chronic illness or disability, and the requirement for long-term caregiving and case management by the family network (Brody, 1985; Felton, 1990; Stephens, Crowther, Hobfoll, & Tennenbaum, 1990). In the sections below, we review a number of the issues that arise during family support and caregiving for an older person to include structural obstacles to effective caregiving, satisfaction with support, caregiver burden, problematic issues in guardianship, and elder abuse.

STRUCTURAL OBSTACLES TO SUPPORT

Even under the best of circumstances, family resources are not unlimited. For many families this will be exacerbated by the kinds of changes in American family life that we noted in Chapter 1 of this volume (an increase in multigenerational families; a declining birth rate that produces fewer siblings to share in parent care; increased life expectancies that extend the duration of parent caregiving involvements; the complexities of divorce, reconstructed, and single-parent families that may stretch the family's responsibilities or undermine its economic base; more women entering the paid work force, and so on (Cantor, 1991).

Families are generally quite adaptable, however, when faced with the need to assume caregiving responsibilities; there are often feelings of mastery, personal reward, and satisfaction in successfully doing so (Horowitz, 1985; Stephens, 1990). Yet, the process of adapting may require a rethinking of the family system and its responsibilities, and a realignment of family roles as the long-term implications of the illness become clear. The family response may also make extraordinary demands on "chosen" members of the family, perhaps because they are the only daughter, live closest to the older parent, or have room in their home for one more soul (Brody, 1985; Stephens, 1990).

Families are likely to differ considerably in how prepared they are to assume these new responsibilities, given their size, structure, history of cohesiveness, coping style, and financial resources. Individual members of the same family are also likely to vary with respect to their level of understanding of the problem and their ability or motivation to help in caring for a given older family member.

Such differences often reflect the obvious factors of finance, geographical proximity, and lack of room for one more in the home. But, they may also reflect an imperfect distribution of information within the family about a parent's specific problems, wishes, or available coping resources. In this connection, Hansson, Nelson, et al. (1990) studied adult children of frail elderly parents to obtain a sense for how families are drawn into the caregiving process. Adult children in this situation appear to follow a conservative, orderly progression in their increasing involvement and intervention. That is, they typically begin thinking and learning about the issues of aging and caregiving generally in response to a health crisis or institutionalization of a parent or other elderly family member or following a serious disruption of a frail parent's support network or coping resources (e.g., a bereavement or financial setback). They may then begin to monitor their parent's health and psychological status more carefully, and subsequently they may become involved. Over 70% of these adult children indicated that they would likely intervene in caregiving or in their parents' decision-making processes. However, their stated criteria for intervention were quite diverse (e.g., if a parent became incompetent or dependent, after a stressful life event such as widowhood, or after significant physical or mental health declines). When they were asked which aspects of their parents' lives they were monitoring more closely these days, their responses were again quite diverse. Approximately 50% of the responses focused on a parent's health, including diet, doctor visits, medications, and so forth. Another 23% focused on their parents' psychological well-being, including emotional status (e.g., loneliness, depression, mood, drinking), maintenance of social relationships, confusion, memory, or stress. Another 23% focused on logistical concerns such as finances, home maintenance, home and neighborhood security, ability to drive safely, or do the grocery shopping.

Children from different families thus appear to adopt very different criteria for deciding whether to intervene in their parents' lives or decision making. Given the complex of variables involved, they are also likely to work through this process with differing levels of information and objectivity. The data of Hansson, Nelson, et al. (1990) data raise one other troubling question, however. Twenty-six percent of the adult children surveyed indicated that they would consider involving themselves in their parents' decision making *only* upon being asked. This "noninterventionist" response may simply reflect a respect for the parent's independence or for the child's past relationship with the parent. Or the parent may have experienced no health crises to date, and the child has not been forced to think about the issue. Nevertheless, it may be important to question the practical implications of waiting to be asked. For example, does the lack of a request for help indicate that the parent's health or support needs are actually being met? Research suggests that we can not make that assumption. Older adults often fail to seek needed health care, perhaps because they don't believe they are ill enough to bother the doctor or because they believe their new symptoms to be natural consequences of the aging process. They may also worry about what they might learn from a doctor visit or about the costs of further tests or hospitalization (Rowe, 1985; Shanas & Maddox, 1985). Finally, as we noted in Chapter 3 of this volume, interactions with health care providers also can be problematic and threatening for older persons.

The manner in which family are drawn into the support process may also reflect the more subtle dynamic of family life. We should not forget, after all, that a family is an assemblage of individuals whose personalities, coping styles, childhoods, and histories of reward and punishment deriving from family membership are likely to differ in important ways.

Each member of the family will have experienced a unique relationship with the particular older person now in need of caregiving, and in later life, some of these relationships may have become strained or antagonistic. The older family member needing support may often have been the source of a conflict that destabilized important family (and potential support) relationships. In one recent study, for example, persons aged 60 and over reported having seriously betrayed 14% of the people in their current social or family network (e.g., by lying, having extramarital affairs, breaking promises, or betraying a confidence; Hansson, Jones, et al., 1990).

Relationships between or among the adult children themselves can also disrupt the family's response to the caregiving needs of a parent. The problem can be seen as one in which individuals (the adult children) must contribute collectively to solve a common problem. Family caregiving may severely stretch the family resources of each of these children. Still, the process generally proceeds amiably as long as each of the contributors feels that the costs and rewards involved have been allocated fairly. Unfortunately, each person in the arrangement will usually have the most detailed information about his/her own contributions to the collective effort. This can lead to a biased cognition that one's own contributions are greater (or outcomes smaller) than that of the others (Lerner, Somers, Reid, & Tierney, 1989). Such cognitions would be expected to strain the collaborative spirit and to undermine its effectiveness. Lerner et al. (1989) studied this phenomenon among adult siblings who were faced with having to provide substantial parent support over the long term. In that study, the subjects reported (on average) feeling that they "contributed more to meeting their parents' needs than did their siblings, had more influence in setting up the present arrangements, felt more trapped by their parents' needs, and felt things would be more fair to everyone if their siblings contributed more . . . " (p. 65).

Finally, families typically do not share the burden of caregiving, acting as an integrated support network. Some family members may feel that contributions of time, housing, or financial resources to assist an elderly parent diminish their ability to meet their responsibilities to their own families and children. The preferred solution, therefore, is often one that minimizes one's own costs, but which also seems "fair." Each child will likely develop a justification for the level of resources he/she is able to commit (Lerner et al., 1989). One member of the family, usually an adult daughter, typically emerges as the primary caregiver (Brody, 1985). Other family members often are willing to assume such responsibility, in serial order, *only* after the previous caregiver has experienced an overwhelming level of stress or burnout and is able to continue no longer (Johnson, 1983). In such cases, then, the elderly family member must endure occasional, involuntary changes of residence. Presumably, each such move would require a renegotiation of mutual expectations, house rules, and equitable living arrangements within the affected household.

At some point, many older persons will require a level of nursing care that is unavailable in the family setting and will enter a long-term care facility. As we noted in Chapter 3, however, close personal relationships are unlikely to form in residential care/nursing home settings. Past friendships and supportive family relationships thus remain important to the patient's adjustment and well-being (Arling, Harkins, & Capitman, 1986; Greene & Monahan, 1982; Harel & Noelker, 1982; Hayslip & Leon, 1992). Unfortunately, however, maintaining contact with one's primary relations from a nursing home can become difficult over time, often requiring a shift in family responsibilities and an increased effort and commitment (Fisher & Tessler, 1986; Greene & Monahan, 1982; Horowitz & Shindelman, 1983). Moreover, it may become more difficult for the older resident to maintain reciprocity and a balance of social exchange within the relationship, potentially weakening ties within the extended family network (Antonucci & Akiyama, 1987). Certain factors, however, do appear to enhance the endurance of one's relational ties when one enters an institution (Bear, 1990). Of particular interest, older persons who have had more frequent contact with members of their network prior to institutionalization tend to remain in closer contact. Also, networks of greater density (i.e., networks whose members are themselves highly interconnected and thus better able to work together on the problem in a team effort) have more enduring ties to the older, institutionalized person. On the other hand, the intensity of one's emotional bonds to members of the network appears not to enhance duration of support ties of the network, suggesting the practical importance of structural support over emotional connections (Bear, 1990).

THE SPECIAL CASE OF SUPPORT
FOR BEREAVED FAMILY MEMBERS

Much is known about the nature of the *individual* bereavement experience, including pattern and course of symptoms over time, risk factors for poor outcome, and processes associated with recovery (e.g., Lund, 1989; Osterweis, Solomon, & Green, 1984; Parkes & Weiss, 1983; Stroebe & Stroebe, 1987; Stroebe et al., 1993). However, recent research has shown that it is also important to consider the *interpersonal* context in which bereavement occurs and the potential impact of bereavement on supportive social networks (O'Bryant & Hansson, in press).

For example, widows often experience a decline in their social or economic status. Also, the deceased spouse may have been the person most often turned to for social support in time of stress, or a primary link to potentially helpful community relationships (Lopata, 1988). In addition, the family's beliefs regarding appropriate sex-role behavior, for example, could limit an older woman's options with respect to employment or remarriage and undermine her efforts to cope independently (Lopata, 1988; Rosenblatt, 1988).

Two major findings are especially interesting in the context of the present chapter and the topic of this book. First, there is now much evidence from the loss and bereavement literature (as there was from research on family caregiving) that some social support efforts work, whereas others do not, and that the latter may do more harm than good (Rosenblatt, 1988; Vachon & Stylianos, 1988; Wortman, Silver, & Kessler, 1993). In this connection, Vachon and Stylianos (1988) proposed that the effectiveness of social support depends on the "goodness of fit" between available support and the individual's needs, given the impact of the loss on both the individual and the involved family network. This viewpoint holds, further, that the best support will be that which is offered in the right amount, at the appropriate time, and by an acceptable source (e.g., one who does not attach strings to the support or demean the recipient). In addition, it will serve the specific support function needed at the time (providing emotional support, a trusted confidante, validation of one's beliefs and feelings, instrumental support, etc.).

Finally, a bereavement can destabilize the family system itself, undermining the very process on which family and social support are based. In this connection, Hansson, Fairchild, Vanzetti, and Harris (1992) recently developed an instrument (the Family Bereavement Inventory; FBI) to assess the impact of bereavement on family systems. The primary factor to emerge in this research involved disintegration and disruption of the family system. Thus, bereaved families who scored higher on the FBI reported that the family had experienced more anger and conflict in the months after the death. They also felt a greater loss in their ability to communicate with one another, and they were more likely to report that the family had lost what it had always stood for; it had begun to drift apart. A second factor emerging from responses to the FBI involved a sense of lost family self-esteem, pride, confidence, and self-respect. A third factor appeared to be a family depression response, involving diminished ability to make decisions or to function productively, and a loss of the family's sense that life remained meaningful and survivable.

Families that scored higher on the FBI (i.e., who reported being more devastated during the 6 months after the death) were those who prior to the death were less cohesive, were experiencing more stress or family conflict, who shared fewer values, interests, and activities. They were also more likely to report marital distress or separations within the family system during the 6 months following the death.

These data suggest that in addition to mourning for the lost person, there is a strong potential element of damage or disruption to the remaining family system. This further suggests that an early task in recovering from bereavement will involve first restabilizing or reconstructing the family support network.

CAREGIVER BURDEN

A huge research literature has now emerged, examining the ways in which caregiving can become a stressor for those providing support (e.g., Pearlin, Mullan, Semple, & Skaff, 1990; Stephens et al., 1990). This research has explored the many conceptual underpinnings of the experience and delineated its consequences for individual caregivers and caregiving networks. At the level of *outcomes,* the more obvious costs to caregivers and their families involve: threats to emotional well-being and physical health; restrictions of privacy, life-style, time, and freedom; reduced attention to outside relationships; and unplanned reallocation of financial resources (Brody, 1985; Cantor, 1983; Horowitz, 1985; Stephens, 1990; Zarit, 1990). Given their context, these kinds of issues are of special concern. For example, a recent national survey profiled the caregivers of noninstitutionalized elderly. Over 35% of the caregivers were themselves aged 65 or older, 30% were poor or near-poor, 33% were in only fair to poor health, and 20% had already been responsible for a disabled older patient for as long as 5 years (Stone et al., 1987).

The potential costs of caregiving are also of consequence outside of the home and family. With increasing numbers of women entering the full-time work force, for example, conflicts arise between caregiving and job responsibilities. A recent study by Scharlach and Boyd (1989) provided an excellent overview of the extent of this problem. In a survey of approximately 1,800 employees of a major employer in southern California, they found 438 of the respondents to be serving in some caregiving role for a person aged 60 or over. The median age of the caregivers was 37 years; approximately two-thirds were women, and 53% indicated having at least one child still at home. Most of the care recipients were women (81%), 78% were parents or in-laws, 11% were grandparents, and the rest were more distant relatives or friends. Much of the support activity involved providing companionship (58%) and help with instrumental needs such as transportation (56%) or housecleaning (30%). Only 8% of the respondents were currently involved in providing more personal care with bathing, feeding, and so forth. Forty-four percent reported that they were the primary caregiver in the situation, and 32% did so without any outside assistance. The majority of respondents reported some degree of emotional (80%), physical (60%), and financial (54%) strain resulting from their caregiver activities.

Caregiving also affected work performance. For example, 73% of caregiver employees in the survey (compared to 49% of non caregiver employees) reported experiencing some interference between work and family responsibilities. Similarly, 37% of the caregivers (but only 23% of noncaregivers) had missed work during the previous 2 months as a result of family responsibilities. Two-thirds of the caregiver sample also reported being interrupted on the job by caregiving-related phone calls, and one-third reported that their duties sometimes made them so tired on the job that it made performance difficult. Twelve percent of caregivers reported that their caregiving responsibilities had been a factor in their choice of their current job.

A diversity of instruments have been developed to assess various aspects of caregiver strain (e.g., Kosberg & Cairl, 1986; Poulshock & Deimling, 1984; Robinson, 1983). These may be useful in identifying caregivers at special risk or those who might benefit from support or counseling efforts. They may be useful also in making decisions about the pending institutionalization of an older adult (Zarit, 1990).

Pearlin et al. (1990) have argued that it is important to view caregiver strain within a broader conceptual model of stress that also accounts for process, stressors specific to the level and type of caregiving required, the context in which caregiving occurs, and potentially compounding personal or social risk factors. Assessments of stressors in their model would thus include measures of the difficulty of the caregiving task (e.g., the recipient's cognitive and functional status, recipient's disruptive behaviors, and caregiver's subjective appraisals of task overload). Assessments of context would delve into the role-strain implications of caregiving (e.g., diminishing role performance in caring for children, on the job, or in maintenance of outside friendships). Assessments of context would also involve measures of family support for the caregiver or family conflict resulting from the disruption of caregiving responsibilities. Assessment of personal or social risk factors would include measures of the caregiver's coping style, self-esteem, mastery, perceived competence to deal with caregiving tasks at hand, and feelings of being trapped in the caregiver role.

Finally, underlying the broad approach to caregiver stress of Pearlin et al. are the affective and symbolic components of the relationship between caregiver and elderly recipient. This relationship will probably change, at some point, from one of mutual exchange and support to one in which unidirectional caregiving becomes the "dominant, overriding component" (p. 583). The altered structure of this relationship, and resulting strain on the emotional bond, appear to be among the core elements of the problem. A large study of caregivers by Cantor (1983), for example, found that the closer the emotional bond, the more strain experienced. In that study, only 53% of caregiver children felt they got along with the dependent parent, compared to 60% of spouse-caregivers, 86% of other relatives involved in caregiving, and 92% of friends or neighbors so involved. Of the children involved in caregiving, only 28% felt that their dependent parent understood them. Many caregivers also appear to feel that other people in general do not understand what their life is like (Barusch, 1988).

A recent study by Walker, Martin, and Jones (1992) is especially informative with respect to the importance of continuing relational factors on the negative outcomes of caregiving (for caregiver and recipient). In this study of older mothers and their caregiver daughters, daughters' negative outcomes fell into three general factors, the pressure of insufficient time, frustration, and a sense of guilt and anxiety that things would not work out. Mothers' negative outcomes involved a sense of feeling guilty and being a burden to the daughter, but also feelings of resentment and anger. All three of the daughters' negative outcomes were lower when they judged their relationship with their mother to be more intimate. Among mothers, feeling the relationship to be more intimate was associated with lowered feelings of resentment or anger. The results of this study suggest that the high costs of a difficult caregiving relationship can be minimized when participants attend to the quality of the relationship itself.

It is also important to remember that caregiving for an older person is often an ongoing commitment, rather than a single event. Schultz, Tompkins, and Rau (1988) examined the implications of this continuing commitment among stroke patients and their caregivers. Both groups had experienced elevated symptoms of depression. At 6 months post-stroke, however, the percentage of patients at risk from depression had decreased from 34% to 25%, whereas the percentage of caregivers at risk remained constant at 34%. Schultz et al. suggest that the caregivers' depression may initially have been a response to the pressures of acute caregiving (1988). Later on, it reflected a growing resignation to the long-term burden of caregiving. It was instructive in this study, also, that after controlling for initial depression levels, follow-up depression scores were higher among caregivers who reported a disruption of their reciprocal confidante relationships and satisfying outside social contacts generally, and among those who felt that their friends and relatives had begun to avoid contact or discussion of their caregiving responsibilities, in part presumably to avoid further burdening the caregiver.

Unfortunately, it is now a common finding that the continuous demands of a caregiving relationship often result in the social isolation of the caregiving dyad from potentially supportive outsiders (Johnson & Catalano, 1983; Hayslip & Leon, 1992). It is also of some concern that problematic emotional and physical health outcomes for the caregiver have been found to be more strongly related to the unavailability of social support than to the actual nature or severity of the patient's impairment (George & Gwyther, 1986).

It is clear, then, that caregiver strain gives rise to a wide variety of potential risks. Foremost among these are that the caregiving needs of a frail elder tend to be long-term, whereas support networks are likely to be chronically stressed, discontinuous, and unpredictable. Such a disparity could seriously impact the quality of care. It could result also in premature failure of the support system and institutionalization of the older person.

SATISFACTION WITH THE CAREGIVING PROCESS

We have seen that the provision of support is possible only within personal or social relationships, which themselves are often problematic. Even the most cohesive and well-meaning of families might expect to be vulnerable to the kinds of "structural" obstacles to support described above. Such constraints make it more difficult for older persons to develop and maintain a diverse network of social resources. In turn, they may be less able to draw upon those particular support resources that might be most appropriate to a given stressful situation (Hobfoll, 1988).

It should not be a surprise that the caregiving situation often spawns conflict, involving as it does two persons with a unique (and often discordant) relational history in a high-stakes undertaking under stressful conditions and with no end in sight. Older persons often find that being dependent on a caregiver, even a close family member, can result in diminished personal control over their lives, broken promises, invasions of privacy, or a frustrating degree of overprotectiveness. Their problems may be viewed to be inconsequential or they may be encouraged to find a way to age more "gracefully" (Norris, Stephens, & Kinney, 1990; Rook, 1984, 1990).

With respect to an older person's psychological well-being, then, the injurious side of a caregiving relationship can outweigh its benefits (Rook, 1984, 1990). Negative social interactions with caregivers also appear to be associated subsequently with problems in being able to perform the basic activities of daily living independently (Norris et al., 1990). These concerns have led some researchers to argue that we should actually shift the focus of our analysis from social support to social relationships (e.g., Stephens & Hobfoll, 1990). Such a reconstrual of the topic might permit a more thorough examination of the positive *and* problematic implications of support efforts for recipient, provider, and family system.

Finally, the family caregiving literature has typically reflected the experience and perceptions of the caregiving family members. Our discussion thus far has also reflected that point of view. But, there is another important voice to be considered—that of the older parent (Troll, 1988). In this connection, Talbot (1990) interviewed older widows (61–85 years of age) regarding any negative aspects of their relationships with their adult children. The goal of the study was to explain a common finding that psychological well-being in old age is related consistently to contact with friends but not to contact with adult children. The most parsimonious explanation may be that supportive relationships and contact with children are an obligation. Supportive efforts in compliance with family obligation might therefore be less likely to impact subjective well-being than if offered through voluntary friendship networks (e.g., Antonucci & Jackson, 1987).

In Talbot's interviews, 49% of the older mothers mentioned a negative side to their relationships with their children, although the nature of the problem took many forms. For example, some mothers simply felt neglected, unappreciated, or dissatisfied with the assistance they received from their children. Others were concerned about becoming a burden on their children. They avoided calling upon their children for help when any other alternative existed. Others felt trapped in a situation of unbalanced emotional dependence. That is, they perceived their dependence on the relationship to be greater than that of their children. Others felt that they were being taken for granted, for example, expected to baby-sit with grandchildren as the price of continued involvement with their children's families. Talbot concluded that such a power imbalance in the relationship could account for the differential value of relationships with children compared to relationships with friends.

ELDER ABUSE

The caregiving relationships described above involve a high potential for feelings of frustration, resentment, and helplessness. It would not be unexpected, therefore, if they occasionally resulted in open conflict and abuse. This has become a matter of increasing concern among older persons, the health professions, and social and governmental agencies. Yet, estimates of elder abuse have been difficult to verify. Research on the topic to date has lacked clear assessment criteria and has relied on small, nonrepresentative victim samples or on reports of officially identified cases. Reliable estimates of the underreporting of abuse by victims or professionals are seldom available.

Nevertheless, the incidence of elder abuse in the United States would appear to be substantial. For instance, a major study of randomly selected persons aged 65 and over in the Boston area recently found an abuse rate of 32 cases per 1,000 persons (Pillemer & Finkelhor, 1988). If these numbers are representative of the population of the United States, then the potential incidence of abuse in this country would be estimated to fall between 701,000 and 1,093,560 cases (Pillemer & Finkelhor, 1988). Of the three types of abuse this study focused on, the rates of physical violence, chronic verbal (psychological) abuse, and neglect were 20/1,000, 11/1,000, and 4/1,000, respectively. Material or financial exploitation was not included in this study, but it will be examined below in connection with recent concerns about abuse in legal guardianship.

In contrast, the Council on Scientific Affairs of the American Medical Association recently concluded, from their analyses of the larger body of existing studies, that the incidence of elder abuse may reach 10% of the population over 65 years of age (Council on Scientific Affairs, 1987). The Council's report introduced AMA Resolution 112, calling upon the Amercian Medical Association to develop diagnostic and treatment guidelines modeled after their guidelines on child abuse and to model state legislation mandating physician reporting.

The data from Pillemer and Finkelhor's study (1988) show that the elderly are most likely to be abused by someone with whom they share housing. As they are more likely to live with a spouse than with their children, the abuser is most often a spouse. In addition, because men are more likely to be living with a spouse, they are at greater risk proportionately (52% of cases in the study) than are women (48% of cases). Because older women outnumber older men in absolute numbers, however, more abuse cases involve women as victims. Older persons and those in poorer health (indicating greater dependency) also appeared to be at greater risk.

A wide variety of other risk factors have been identified as well, many of them reflecting the complexity of family relationships. Kosberg (1988) summarized this research in an attempt to identify the characteristics of the older person or family that increase the risk of abuse. For example, *high-risk elderly* appear to include women (because of their numbers), the very old (whose assistance needs are more demanding), those who contribute to family conflict (e.g., because of disruptive behavior or alcohol problems), and those with preexisting conflicts with the caregiver child. *High-risk caregivers* appear to include persons who have their own emotional problems or pathologies, who lack caregiving experience or an understanding of age-related changes in cognitive or physical functioning, have unrealistic expectations for the relationship, are undergoing financial stress, or are socially isolated. Finally, there also appear to be a number of characteristics that place the caregiving *family system at greater risk*. These factors generally reflect the existence of external family stressors, a lack of family coping resources, and the absence of family determination to persevere in taking care of its own. Thus, families at risk of abuse more frequently appear to involve a caregiver who did not volunteer, who has little integrated support from other family members, or for whom the addition of the elderly care recipient results in serious overcrowding of the home, loss of privacy, or inconvenience. In addition, families at risk are likely to have preexisting financial problems or a preference that the elderly person be institutionalized rather than placed in their home. Finally, the caregiving family itself may be experiencing conflict (e.g., marital conflict or distress), or may already be burdened (e.g., with an alcoholic adult or a chronically ill child), making it difficult to stretch family coping resources or establish caregiving priorities.

Of particular concern, abused older persons and their families are often socially isolated (Kosberg, 1988). They are less likely to have access to social or community support services that could aid them in times of stress and be in a position to notice and report instances of obvious abuse. This would seem a critical point, given the conspiracy of silence surrounding elder abuse in families (U.S. Congress, House Select Committee on Aging, 1980). For a variety of reasons, only about one-sixth of elder abuse cases are actually reported (Kosberg, 1988). A common reason is that in our culture the family's life is private; by tradition, prescribed rights to family independence preclude outside interference. Also, it is common for elderly family members to be home-bound or bedridden, so their maltreatment may not be noticed by others. In addition, elderly persons may hesitate to report their abusers, owing to feelings that it is a private affair, or to a concern that the alternative to this family situation might be something even worse, such as institutionalization.

In response, most states have now enacted legislation mandating that physicians report suspected cases of elderly abuse (Shapiro, 1992). Unfortunately, statutes are not uniform in their definition of prohibited behavior or in their specification of protected populations. Moreover, they often provide no follow-through. Many states provide for reporting and investigation but not for delivery of services (Daniels, Baumhover, & Clark-Daniels, 1989). Also, many states have failed to fund need-ed agencies to investigate reports of abuse or to provide protective services (Hagedorn, 1990).

It is also a concern that physicians are often uncomfortable with these new reporting laws, as evidenced by a recent study of 156 Alabama physicians (Daniels et al., 1989). In this survey, only 60% of physicians believed that an experienced clinician could accurately diagnose elder abuse. Only 17% felt that AMA-provided definitions of what constitutes abuse were clear-cut. Seventy-nine percent felt that they could probably better handle suspected cases of abuse themselves, rather than reporting them to authorities. Many physicians also had personal reasons for being hesitant to report abuse. For example, 49% expressed the belief that their anonymity would not be protected. Thirty-six percent worried that they would be required to spend considerable time in court appearances. Such concerns clearly have the potential to undermine the intent of mandatory reporting legislation.

GUARDIANSHIP ISSUES

A final issue touching on family abuse of the elderly involves legal guardianship. It is now common for family members to petition for full guardianship of an elderly parent if they sense that their parent needs protection beyond the usual domains of caregiving. There are between 300,000 and 400,000 elderly persons now under guardianship (Bayles & McCartney, 1987).

Full guardianship in most states includes decision-making authority over personal, financial, and estate affairs. Thus, affected older individuals lose their rights to live where they wish or with whom, to marry or divorce, or engage a lawyer or physician of their choice. Here, also, widespread concerns (and reports) regarding potential abuse have recently drawn considerable attention both from legislators and the press (e.g., Bayles & McCartney, 1987; U.S. Select Committee on Aging, 1987).

A recent analysis of guardianship proceedings in the states of Washington and Ohio provides a number of insights regarding the vulnerability of older persons who are the target of such proceedings. This analysis also reveals a lack of safeguards for their rights and preferences (Bulcroft, Kielkopf, & Tripp, 1991). These are presented below:

1. Full and permanent guardianship is typically awarded, failing to take into account the possibility of an older adult ever regaining competence (e.g., after rehabilitation from a stroke).
2. The median estate in a guardianship is approximately $52,000. The underlying purpose of most petitions appears to be the preservation of that estate, especially when family interests are threatened (e.g., if the parent wishes to give the money to friends or charity rather than to the children). It is also fascinating, in this context, that, whereas the vast majority of hands-on caregivers are female, the majority of petitioners for guardianship are male and that in about 50% of cases, there is some controversy over who should become guardian.
3. Guardianship decisions typically do not reflect reliable or valid assessments of the competence of the older adult, or acknowledgment of the potential for improvement of such competence with improved health. Instead, courts tend to rely on petitioner testimony and physician reports that may be vague, out of date, or poorly documented. In most states there exists no requirement for periodic follow-up reviews of competence and no mechanism for restoration of rights. A related analysis of court documents by the Associated Press discovered a multitude of additional concerns (Bayles & McCartney, 1987). In their review of 2,200 cases representing all 50 states, 30% of all files involved no medical evidence, 49% of the elderly persons being reviewed did not attend their hearing, and 25% of the case files provided no evidence that a formal hearing was actually conducted. The Associated Press concluded that many older persons don't even know about

the proceedings until they learn they have become wards of the court. Finally, once guardianship decisions are completed, the guardian's performance with regard to managing and safeguarding the older person's financial assets is seldom audited, given scarce state resources for enforcement.

4. Few older persons ever legally challenge guardianship petitions, although they sometimes try to oppose the process informally. They almost never engage their own legal counsel, and they appear unwilling to challenge family members, for many of the same reasons that they are unwilling to report physical abuse. That is, they are likely to be physically frail and require caregiving, may be embarrassed about the nature of the proceedings, are perhaps too loyal to family members, or they fear retaliation and the loss of future family support.

Also entangled in the ethical problems of guardianship are the involved attorneys. The legal profession has begun to explore the ethical issues and to search for safeguards (Donaldson, 1991). This can be difficult, however, owing to the overlapping and potentially conflicted client relationships possible in guardianship cases. For example, the attorney often will have had previous client relationships with members of the family (rather than the elderly person who is the subject of the guardianship proceedings). The attorney may also have become involved in the current proceedings at the request of family members and is often compensated by these family members. Under such circumstances, who is the client? Whose rights come first? What is the attorney's obligation to meet privately with the elderly family member to assure the elder's needs, wishes, and autonomy? Where the attorney's participation constitutes multiple representation, what rules or ethics guide disclosure of confidential information between parties? How can attorneys fairly serve the best interests of both parties?

As in other areas of family law, attorneys should be able to help families deal with the practicalities of guardianship without violating the rights and autonomy of the elder. In particular, model codes of professional responsibility should address the ethical and facilitative role that attorneys could play in helping families of the frail elderly to think through these issues prior to the onset of any serious disability or loss of capacity (Donaldson, 1991).

In this chapter and in Chapter 3, we have examined the kinds of obstacles faced by families and social support networks as they deal with the needs of their older members. These obstacles involve considerable complexity and may test the limits of a network's stability, efficacy, or integrity. During the extended process of caregiving for the elderly, families, friends, and more formal support systems can be seen at their best, and unfortunately, at their worst. Usually, however, they are seen to muddle through, providing what they can, as best they can, experiencing considerable burden.

In the next chapter, we examine these issues from the viewpoint of the older person being served by a support network. We propose a model of the related interpersonal contexts of old age, and of the challenges to be faced within each context by an older person who would hope to impact the process.

CHAPTER 5

THE INTERPERSONAL CONTEXTS OF OLD AGE

In the preceding chapters, we explored broadly the nature of human aging, associated demands for coping and adaptation, and the many ways in which successful adaptation depends on one's personal relationships. It became evident during the process that supportive relationships in later life are immensely complex. Their capacity to match an older adult's needs may be enhanced or undermined in many ways.

Relationships, support networks, and their functions often become less predictable with age. As we begin to experience greater age-related illness and disability, our needs for assistance become more complex and long-term. Yet, the inner circle of our networks is also aging and itself changing. Caregiving becomes increasingly formal as the burden is shared with outsiders. Relationships and their support functions are less likely to be initiated or controlled by the older person, and decisions begin to be made by persons or entities further from the locus of the individual. Cantor (1979, 1991) argues that these relationships should be viewed within a systems model of "social care." The social care system is organized hierarchically, with the closest, informal kin networks being activated first. Subsequently, support is sought from neighbors and friends, more formal community networks, voluntary and service agencies, and government entities should the more immediate kin networks be overwhelmed. The various components of the social care system occasionally overlap in function, however, and an older person may be involved with several of them at one time. Cantor (1991) holds that "such assistance augments individual competency and mastery of the environment rather than increasing dependency" (p. 337). Within limits, this is probably true.

However, in later life the relationships on which we depend for support can also become less accessible, strained, mismatched to needs, and interpersonally problematic. At such times, the relational competencies an older adult brings to each situation can make a difference, allowing some older persons to deal more effectively with potentially supportive others, even (and perhaps especially) under difficult circumstances.

We discuss relational competence in considerable detail in later chapters. However, it is first necessary to try to conceptualize the relational situations we have encountered thus far, with respect to the demands they place on an individual's social coping resources. In this chapter, therefore, we provide a number of integrative analyses of the interpersonal contexts of old age.

For purposes of the first analysis, we have selected many of the interpersonal situations encountered in earlier chapters of the book. Table 5.1 arrays these situations on an age-related continuum, ranging from those situations in which the older person still maintains a high degree of personal autonomy—to those in which the individual has reached the point of substantial dependency on social or caregiving relationships. The analysis takes into account a person's changing competencies. It also takes into account changing needs for social resources (e.g., for companionship, support, security, involvement, stimulation, or inclusion) and changing interpersonal circumstances across the later years. This analysis then goes to one of the underlying issues of interpersonal aging, our ability to manage social transition, given diminishing competence and increasing vulnerability. It sets the stage for a parallel analysis of relational competence.

The reader will note that many of the core tasks of relating remain important across the interpersonal contexts illustrated in Table 5.1. These include accessing, maintaining, and building relationships, negotiating rules and asserting one's rights, establishing structure, and contributing to the stability of the relationship or family unit. But, as an older person progresses through the situations characteristic of later ages, the implications of changing competence and a changing support environment become evident and may require an alteration of one's goals or strategies.

Table 5.1 illustrates the changing nature of social interaction in later life. Older persons generally appear to become more dependent on support relationships, which are likely to become more strained, unpredictable, and formal over time. As we have seen, however, a number of additional social and family dynamics may further constrain the older adult's efficacy in mobilizing social coping resources. These

TABLE 5.1. Relational Situations Generally Ordered by Remaining Autonomy

New situation	Relational challenge
MAINTAINING CURRENT STATUS AND LEVEL OF AUTONOMY	
Diminished occupational status, options	Broaden social networks and interests to compensate; assume new (generative) roles in work organization (sharing, mentoring, etc.)
Maintaining level of commitment/contribution to family	Adjust to shifting family roles, reduced demands by children; remain adaptive, flexible regarding new demands (e.g., divorced children returning home, family emergencies)
Friendships lost to death, retirement, relocation, etc.	Replace lost relationships, social roles; find ways to develop secondary relationships into primary
Isolating consequences of unemployment, retirement	Overcome embarrassment, stigma; broadly call on social networks for assistance, contacts, new opportunities; find new sense of purpose, new (nonoccupational) sources of meaning, self-worth
Unsafe, problem neighborhoods	Establish compensating community networks, services
First interactions with formal support systems (e.g., medical, governmental)	Establish contact with "gatekeepers," relationships with professionals; monitor and evaluate services; assert rights
Confronted with agist stereotypes	Accurately communicate needs to others (e.g., to physicians who may attribute physical symptoms to "usual" aging, or to family who may want to prematurely intervene in affairs)
Bereavement	Restabilize family system; recruit emotional, health, financial support; overcome constraints to exercising coping options
Living alone	Compensate for built-in support system
Increasing frailty	Adjust to increasing isolation; assertively seek services
Onset of serious health problems	Diagnosis and treatment become complex, involve more systems, require one to negotiate, coordinate, and monitor efforts of numerous, multidisciplinary professionals and caregivers
Complex support needs	Need to manage efforts of others to obtain support that matches one's needs (e.g., right form of support, by most effective source, minimizing strings, conflicts, inequities)

(continued)

TABLE 5.1. *(Continued)*

New situation	Relational challenge
Intervention by adult children	Establish ground rules with 70% of children who will intervene when *they* believe needed; get the attention of the 25% likely to *do nothing until asked*
Becoming dependent on caregivers, supporters, and networks	Understand perspective and situation of caregivers, find ways to overcome troubled personal history with caregiver; assert own needs, rights, roles; deal with invasions of privacy, frustrated feelings, conflict, caregiver attempts to intervene in your relationships with health, financial, or legal professionals
Family conflict about equitable allocation of caregiver duties	Understand that children are unlikely to know facts of others' involvements, will want to contribute their fair share, but will likely overestimate the value of their own contribution; someone must clarify, organize, mediate negotiations
Confronted with health/home care staff	Overcome mistrust or miscommunication caused by differences in social class, race, age
Caregiver strain, breakdown	Often results in neglect, abuse, or decision to institutionalize; older recipient must find ways to recognize, moderate, minimize, and offset strain
Caregiver burnout results in a "hand-off"	Need to manage transition; negotiate new relationships and household routines, find ways to support new caregiver relationship
Neglectful or abusive family caregivers	May be one's only housing option, so cannot leave; may be afraid to report abuse because of embarrassment, belief that family life is private, fear that abuser (child/spouse) will be punished or abandon elder to an institution; so must try to deal with family member who may have own emotional problems, stress, or pathology, or who lacks understanding of age-related change and has unrealistic expectations for elder's abilities; or with family system that lacks coping resources, is overcrowded and inconvenienced, may be experiencing destabilizing marital conflict, and may be socially isolated and not monitored or supported in relationship with elder
Threatened by guardianship proceedings	Prior to becoming vulnerable, must minimize risk of abuses of guardianship law and relationship; establish own relationships with phy- *(continued)*

TABLE 5.1. (*Continued*)

New situation	Relational challenge
	sicians, attorneys, friends, trusted family members; draw the line between embarrassment and need; communicate wants, needs, preferences to family and others while still competent and independent; invest in such protections and relationships while they are still available
Entering senior housing	Senior housing environment is not a dominant source of supportive relationships, so must maintain contact and negotiations with family; must deal with "barriers" to new friendships (e.g., frailer residents cannot keep up reciprocal support exchanges, so are often excluded; older and frailer residents are subject to discrimination on basis of health status)
Decision making about institutionalization	Decisions often reflect family stress and circumstances as well as elder's health status and nursing needs; for every person in a nursing home, two of similar disability status are cared for at home; find out how to (1) defer institutionalization for the wrong reasons, and (2) ensure own participation in decision making
Entering the nursing home/institutional care	Coming to terms with standardized routine and living space, power of nursing staff to designate treatment or housing options (and potential abuse of such power), poorly trained staff who don't know much about you and may not share your background, values, race, gender, socioeconomic status or marital status; given few friends or confidants among residents, how to maintain contact with primary relationships on the outside; given distances involved, difficulty of maintaining reciprocal social exchange relationships with outside family and friends, and the need for outside family and friends to also focus on their own families and lives

FULL DEPENDENCY

issues become critical as an older individual experiences diminishing competencies and successive levels of dependency. The concern is one of person–environment fit. A number of these dynamics are summarized in Table 5.2.

In this connection, Lawton and Simon (1968) noted that older

TABLE 5.2. Relational/Caregiving Dynamics with Age

Friendships	Networks narrow as a result of retirement, relocation, deaths; loss of income, health or independence result in inability to maintain contact, reciprocity
Convoys of support	Relationships and networks evolve and change over time, varying in size, complexity, and function in response to normative family and occupational cycle, and to individual's needs
Role contraction	Social roles contract becoming empty of meaning and function; reduced demands for social performance; social inclusion more dependent on protocol, tradition, goodwill
Modernity	Society has become more voluntaristic; older person must take initiative; not the society elderly person grew up in
Stereotyping	Older adults' problems are discounted/attributed to "natural" aging process; less rigorous diagnostic/treatment efforts; disinterest by professionals in less convenient older patients
Changing families	Changing capacity of aging family; diminished and stressed networks; increased divorce, geographic mobility, fewer siblings; older, frailer caregivers; multigenerational caregiver burdens; family–work conflict
Family decision making	Conservative progression of family being drawn into intervention situations
Progressive networks	Support/caregiving typically assumed first by immediate family; subsequent aid sought from extended family, community, formal agencies, and broader societal support/health care structures
Support "match"	Difficulty of support fit; right amount, right time, right function; no strings, etc.
Social exchange	Gradually diminished capacity to contribute to social-exchange underpinnings of friendships and family interactions

persons who are less competent in terms of their physical health, psychological, or social competence have a narrower range of adaptability to environmental press. They termed such vulnerability "environmental docility." Research on environmental press has generally supported this contention, for example, finding less competent older adults to be more immediately distressed when housing or neighborhood conditions deteriorate and become less supportive or secure (Lawton, 1980; Morgan et al., 1984). Similarly, a deteriorating, less supportive or secure social (or family) environment could more immediately become problematic for less competent older persons. That is, the environmental docility concept may also have heuristic value in understanding individual differences in coping with problematic social environments. In particular, older persons who are experiencing successive levels of dependency on supportive others should be less able to accommodate those social or caregiving support efforts that are a "poor fit" to current needs. Such individuals would likely have a reduced range of adaptability to social or caregiving situations that are ineffective, strained, or otherwise problematic. They are the candidates for premature institutionalization or abuse.

AN INTEGRATIVE MODEL OF INTERPERSONAL CONTEXTS IN OLD AGE

A great many factors thus interact to determine the availability and efficacy of an older person's social and family support systems. These factors include (1) the individual's functional status and independence, (2) the likely nature of support involvement by family and others, (3) the nature and competency of the support network, (4) "relational coping" demands on the older individual, and (5) the relational competencies of the older individual. We have tried to conceptualize the likely interactions of these factors in Table 5.3.

For purposes of analysis in Table 5.3, we have divided the transition to dependency in later life into seven phases. Our purpose here is not to establish a "stage model" of adult dependency but simply to acknowledge significant milestones in the progression, so that the interpersonal context and implications may be further explored. In fact, we would expect (consistent with assumptions of the life-span developmental orientation: Baltes, 1987) that for any given individual, the trajectory of change with respect to dependency will reflect both cumulative and discontinuous factors, may be multidirectional, will probably involve a blend of losses and gains, and that many such changes may be modifiable or reversible. Thus, an individual recovering from an illness or a bereavement might also recover a degree of independence from supportive social networks.

However, there would appear to be limits to the developmental reserves of older adults. Experimental research generally finds, for example, that while interventions are often able to improve lost function (e.g., cognitive or physical), older adults typically gain proportionately less from intervention than do younger adults (see review in Baltes, 1987). It seems appropriate, therefore, to view the

TABLE 5.3. Interpersonal Contexts in Old Age

Phase of dependency	Likely nature of support	Network status/ competence	Relational coping demands
Healthy young-old, independent	Minimal, voluntary, "when asked"	Young, healthy, competent	Healthy aging; socially integrated; still a contributor
Marginally independent, needs some help	Conservative family help; early thoughts about long-term needs	Spouse/caregiver aging, kids involved with own families	Access, construct, nurture network
Requires some caregiving	Negotiations among family about caregiver responsibilities	Learning caregiving roles; uncertainty about roles, equitable distribution of responsibilities	Clarify, assert needs, preferences, ground rules; negotiate exchange relationships
Requires full-time caregiving	Probable family involvement; some professional involvement	Caregiver strain, turnover, costs of burden to family	Exhibit willingness to be helped, patience, gratitude, flexibility, understanding of caregiver's situation; balance burden with rewards
Requires supportive housing or nursing care	Often involuntary relocation; separation from friends, family; few new relationships	Reduced contact with family, friends; more contact with staff; fundamental change in functions of support (medical/caregiving); staff untrained, poorly paid, stressed	Make new friends; increase family contact; understand practical demands of institutional life; yet assert needs and rights; open lines of communication with staff; ease burden on others
Institutionalized	Dependence on staff; few relationships; diminished physical/social competence		
Marginally competent to make decisions	Family involvement/negotiations; learning about options, guardianship	Demands on judgment, ethics of family members as they make decisions for elderly member	Little to be done now; likely marginally competent; dependent on good will and judgment of relationships built earlier

first column of Table 5.3 as a typical progression of successive levels of dependency.

We might make the same point about the second and third columns of Table 5.3. Given families and support networks vary greatly in their preparedness, willingness, and competence to assume support responsibilities. These columns are also intended to portray what is likely to be happening at the various stages of the *typical* family cycle. Column 2 illustrates the evolving nature of likely support in later life. Early on, support is not likely to be an issue; family views on the topic are likely to be diverse, unorganized, and uninformed. In response to health or life events, however, the family typically begins to think, learn, and organize around the issues. Simultaneously, the family network is aging and changing. At some point, questions arise regarding the family network's continued ability to deal with successive levels of case management or caregiving, and more formal solutions are sought (nursing care, housing options, etc.).

Of central importance in Table 5.3 are our assumptions in the fourth column, regarding the kinds of relational coping demands facing an older adult at each phase of dependency. Here, again, there will be considerable overlap; for example, the need to clarify and assert one's needs could become important at any stage, given the nature and competence of the available support network. In this column, however, we have tried to anticipate the relational coping tasks most central at each stage.

In the next chapter, we provide a precise theoretical and measurement model for the construct of relational competence and predictions regarding which specific components of relational competence are likely to be most important at each stage of dependency. We would expect large individual differences in the likelihood that older persons will exhibit relational competencies appropriate to the demands of the interpersonal context of their current stage of dependency. Further, we would expect those who are more relationally competent to be more able to access or construct support networks when needed and to be more sensitive to the status and maintenance needs of the network. They should also be more adaptable in the face of a support network that is strained, interpersonally problematic, or simply a poor fit or match to their current needs. We have attempted to illustrate these expectations in Figure 5.1.

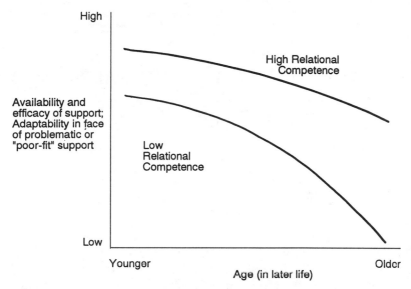

FIGURE 5.1. The efficacy of one's support networks is expected to be a function of the older recipient's age and degree of relational competence. Older persons with greater relational competence should generally experience fewer losses of independence and be more adaptable when faced with strained or "poor-fit" support resources.

THEORY AND MEASUREMENT OF RELATIONAL COMPETENCE

I t was our early work on the interpersonal correlates of significant life problems that led us to first propose the construct of relational competence. We found across several studies a variety of interpersonal characteristics and beliefs that had quite similar patterns of association with other phenomena. For example, in a study of diabetics we found negative mood states and beliefs about control of the diabetes to be associated with indices of positive relational functioning, such as assertiveness and beliefs that the family cooperated with treatment (Carpenter, Hansson, Rountree, & Jones, 1983). We also found that these variables accounted for the strong association between social satisfaction and diabetes outcomes. That is, relational competence variables predicted diabetes outcomes in the same way as knowing about one's overall satisfaction with relationships. Thus, we hypothesized that relational competence was an important determinant of functioning, perhaps by contributing to positive relationships. Specifically, successful relationships yield many benefits (including many that are not interpersonal), but successful relationships depend on relational competence (Jones, 1985).

A similar convergence of such variables was found in a cross-cultural examination of the correlates of loneliness (Jones, Carpenter, & Quintana, 1985). For example, although conceptually distinct, we found high correlations among assertiveness, lack of shyness, lack of social anxiety, masculinity (instrumental competence), need for achievement, and self-esteem. In fact, this study helped highlight the fact that "competence" variables tended to go together. The cross-cultural data, then, helped us initially determine what kinds of interpersonal variables were most likely to fit our general concept of relational competence.

About this time we offered a general definition of relational competence, oriented around the functions these competencies might serve. Thus, relational competence was viewed to involve those "characteristics of the individual that facilitate the acquisition, development, and maintenance of mutually satisfying relationships" (Hansson, Jones, & Carpenter, 1984, p. 273). Drawing upon the loneliness and shyness literature, we proposed a variety of mechanisms by which such competence could partially account for the development of social support and for the connections between support and various health and adjustment outcomes. We anticipated that a broad range of relational skills could eventually be incorporated into the construct of relational competence and that such skills would likely serve four functions. First, they would encourage individuals to conceptualize relationships positively, as a coping resource for other important life functions. Second, they would aid in constructing satisfying relationships. Third, they would enable a person to access relationships, especially in time of need. Finally, they would enhance the maintenance of important relationships so as to make them more meaningful, accessible, and enduring. Examples of characteristics and interpersonal behaviors that might serve each function are shown in Table 6.1.

Although the definition was intentionally broad at the beginning, certain boundaries were established. First, the model narrows relational competence to characteristics that serve one's relationships, increasing the chance that the individual will benefit. Thus, behaviors that simply occur in a social context, such as communication competence (cf. Spitzberg & Cupach, 1989), might not be included. Second, the focus is on the individual, rather than the partner or dyad. And third, relational competence refers to characteristics of that individual. It is certainly appropriate to study social transactions, but that is not our intent for relational competence, which we limit to attributes of the individual. Similarly, one might appropriately study specific behaviors, but we believe that more will be learned by examining more global, enduring characteristics.

THE TWO-COMPONENT MODEL
OF RELATIONAL COMPETENCE

Our initial definition generated a number of interesting studies, but the broad definition yielded measurement strategies that were so varied as to be difficult to compare. For example, Carpenter (1985) operationalized relational competence with three personality characteristics—shyness, interpersonal sensitivity, and self-consciousness. Hansson

TABLE 6.1. The Functions of Relational Competence

Function	Examples of enduring attributes that serve the function	Examples of beliefs and social behaviors that result from the attribute
Conceptualizing	Self-confidence	Beliefs that others will like and accept you and that you can win them over
Constructing	Friendliness	Approaching others in a positive, open, and receptive manner
Accessing	Trust	Acting in ways that tell others you think they are good and will help you
Maintaining	Perspective-taking	Being inclined to view problems from the other person's point of view

(1986a), used an adaptation of the Bem Sex Role Inventory, defining dimensions of instrumentality and sensitivity. Davis and Oathout's (1987) approach emphasized empathy. Hogg and Heller (1990) took exception to the trait approach, recommending a greater focus on particular task demands and specific skills, in a more behavioral tradition.

Most early work, then, measured rather traditional personality attributes as representative of relational competence. Not only was this successful, but a focus on enduring attributes of the person matched our definition of relational competence. Whereas the more molecular measurement approach of Hogg and Heller (1990) seems an appropriate alternative, increased behavioral specificity would likely make any instrument more situation- and population-specific.

The next step, then, was to propose a structure for the relevant attributes that could guide us to more consistent assessment of relational competence. The emphasis on four functions, though useful, did not provide that structure. Even though relational competence serves these functions, it is evident that many social competencies serve more than one function. For example, assertiveness might serve two functions, relationship constructing and relationship accessing. In recognition of this, both Hansson (1986a) and Davis and Oathout (1987) redefined relational competence somewhat, emphasizing two primary components. Davis and Oathout specifically suggested that one set of attributes is most useful for constructing and accessing relationships, whereas another set is most useful for maintaining relationships. A number of existing lines of evidence also argued for a two-component model (we discuss these below). Thus, we adopted such a model (Carpenter, 1987) and describe it here.

Initiation

The first component, labeled *Initiation,* includes those skills most relevant for initiating, controlling, and making demands upon relationships. They likely help one take charge in social situations and may serve as direct coping skills, especially for *problem-focused* coping (coping behaviors that seek to remove the source of stress). These skills tend to be those tangibly valued in society and are often associated with success and adjustment. Relevant attributes could include, for example, self-confidence, assertiveness, social interest, communication skills, likability, and extraversion.

Enhancement

The second component, labeled *Enhancement,* includes skills for enhancing and maintaining relationships, thereby making them more accessible, useful, satisfying, and enduring. They involve investing in relationships and often serve the needs of one's partner or partners in relationships. Although enhancement skills are socially valued, tangible rewards are less evident. These skills appear less likely to serve directly as coping behaviors and often have costs of vulnerability and self-sacrifice associated with them. They may, however, serve as coping resources by making relationships more accessible and useful; hence, their benefits might be largely realized indirectly through enduring relationships, such as in marriage. Relevant attributes could include, for example, empathy, altruism, social awareness, listening skills, and flexibility.

Examples of attributes falling into the two domains are provided in Table 6.2. For most interpersonal variables, placement of the attributes is fairly obvious, and empirical data gives support. However, a few important social constructs are not so easily placed. For example, likability, friendliness, and openness seem relevant to both domains. Similarly, self-disclosure and flexibility are hard to place (e.g., simply being disclosing may help neither the development nor maintenance of relationships if the disclosure is not appropriate to the situation).

RELATED CONSTRUCTS

Interest in interpersonal competence has a long history with many branches. Examples of early work include social intelligence (e.g., Thorndike, 1920), focusing on mental processing and social informa-

TABLE 6.2. Aligning Common Personality Attributes with the Two-Component Model of Relational Competence

Initiation domain	Enhancement domain
Relational attributes	
Extraversion	Agreeableness
Sociability	Need affiliation
Shyness (negative)[a]	Dependence (mild levels)
Social anxiety (negative)[a]	Empathy
Self-confidence	Altruism[a]
Control	Interpersonal sensitivity[a]
Dominance[a]	Intimacy[a]
Assertiveness[a]	Trust[a]
Expressive skills	Love
Social interest	Nurturance
Self-promotion	Self-sacrificing
Narcissim (moderate levels)	Perspective taking[a]
	Listening skills
	Social awareness
Mostly nonrelational attributes that are likely correlates	
Instrumental competence[a]	Reflectiveness
Need achievement	Impulsivity (negative)
Self-esteem	Honesty
Energy	Internalization of societal norms
Enthusiasm	Social responsibility
Range of interests	

[a]Attributes selected for inclusion in the Relational Competence Scale.

tion, and social competence (e.g., Doll, 1935), initially examining mental deficiency, and maladaptive social functioning. Spitzberg and Cupach (1989) reviewed the diversity of work on the topic and concluded that there are myriad perspectives and approaches. They suggested that the numerous conceptual and methodological frameworks have led to some confusion but also to richness and varied application.

Spitzberg and Cupach (1989) offered a broad definition of interpersonal competence, "the process whereby people effectively deal with each other" (p. 6). Alternative definitions could include, for example, the appearance of competence in a particular relationship or in relationships generally (e.g., Spitzberg & Hecht, 1984), or adequacy of behavior in interpersonal transactions (e.g., Burns & Farina, 1984). Clearly, these approaches are intended to examine much the same phenomena. And yet each makes decisions regarding what is studied (process, transaction, ability) at what level (specific behaviors to broad dispositions) and from what perspective (actor, observer, or dyad).

Also, some value judgment is usually implied, such that some behaviors are competent, right, or preferred, and others are not, although these judgments may be context-specific or more absolute.

In fact, the varied approaches that are typically included under general terms like interpersonal competence, social competence, and social skill are often not clearly articulated. Thus, the terms remain necessarily vague (Conger & Conger, 1982; Spitzberg & Cupach, 1989). It is largely for this reason that we chose to propose a new term, *relational competence,* which could be broad and encompassing, but maintain sufficient specificity to provide clear direction and meaning. As will be seen, the approach still falls well within the field of inter-personal competence.

Leary's Interpersonal Circle and Related Approaches

Leary (1957) was one of the first to propose a two-dimensional model of interpersonal functioning. He described a circumplex model of relational behavior, with dimensions of dominance–submission and love–hate at the orthogonal, primary axes (see Box 6.1). Although largely intuitive at the time, considerable empirical support has emerged for the general approach (cf. Horowitz & Vitkus, 1986). Leary's Interpersonal Circle includes 16 distinctive, behaviorally defined segments ordered around the two dimensions, although his writings focus primarily on eight labeled pairs. Leary appeared less interested in the factors or primary axes than in the separate categories, but the similarities to the two-component model of relational competence are obvious.

Other descriptions of interpersonal behavior and functioning support such a two-part approach. Examination of reviews from various theoretical orientations (e.g., Bierman, 1969; Carson, 1969; Horowitz & Vitkus, 1986; Wiggins, 1982), reveals substantial similarity across most models. Some theories, for example, label the dimensions control and affiliation or label the continuum ends dominance/submission and nurturance/rejection, but the underlying constructs are quite similar across models.

When first developing the two-component model of relational competence, Carpenter (1987) assumed that the approach would readily parallel the work of Leary and others. However, there do appear to be a few modest distinctions. For example, much past work emphasizes behavior classification. In fact, the circumplex approach is perhaps most valuable for understanding the relationships among various interpersonal behaviors, with less attention to why such behaviors occur, how consistent patterns develop, and what impact they have on functioning. Hence, attention focuses more on the circumplex segments

LEARY'S CIRCUMPLEX

Circumplex models organize related characteristics around a circle, in which attributes that tend to go together are placed close to one another, attributes that are opposites are placed opposite to one another, and attributes that are uncorrelated are placed at 90° angles. Because a circle is a two-dimensional object, this approach allows characterization of a model of two independent (uncorrelated) dimensions.

The circle is placed so that one dimension is vertical, with one extreme at the top and its opposite at the bottom. The other dimension, uncorrelated with the first, is horizontal, with one extreme at the left and the opposite extreme at the right. Portions of the circle not at these poles indicate some combination of the two dimensions. Thus, the upper-left portion of the circle reflects attributes that are high on the vertical dimension and low on the horizontal dimension.

The circumplex model can be used to organize attributes (or people, behaviors, relationships, and so forth) by the extent to which they include elements of the two dimensions. This "mapping" is easily done by correlating a measure of the attribute with measures of the two dimensions; the correlations represent vectors in x and y space from the circle's center. For example, correlations of .6 with the vertical axis and $-.3$ with the horizontal axis places the mapped item in the upper-left quadrant. Appearing about midway between the center of the circle and the edge, the mapped attribute is "moderately" similar to that reflected by the circumplex dimensions.

Leary developed a circumplex model of interpersonal functioning, with power (dominance versus submission) and affiliation (love versus hate) dimensions. Various combinations of these two dimensions make up the other segments of the circle. Thus, those high in both power and affiliation (upper right part of the circle) might be described as responsible or helpful.

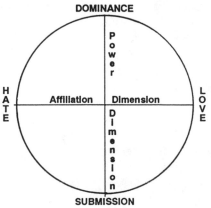

BOX 6.1. Circumplex models and Leary's Interpersonal Circle.

than on the underlying dimensions. However, some (e.g., Wiggins & Broughton, 1984) have specifically characterized the ways of relating as traits, and a number of the relational models imply as much.

Another possible distinction comes from viewing relevant attributes as competencies, something that earlier models tended not to do. For example, even though Leary's naming (e.g., love–hate) implies a value judgment, he remained more neutral in his descriptions. Thus, those high on Love might be described as effusive, doting, and over-conventional, as well as friendly. In contrast, describing the two dimensions as skills, as in relational competence, puts a different twist to the attributes.

Finally, important features of Leary's model are complementarity and purpose. From his perspective, the purpose of specific behaviors is to invite complementary reactions from others, largely in an effort to achieve security in relationships by making them consistent, predictable, and self-serving. In contrast, the model of relational competence is less concerned with purpose and specific reactions from others. A general, single-minded purpose—to promote positive relationships—is inherent in the formulation of relational competence, but little is implied beyond that.

Five-Factor Models of Personality

Early formulations of personality varied widely in their attention to social functioning, but the emphasis was often not on interpersonal skills and attributes relevant to relationship building. In contrast, such characteristics hold a prominent position in recent conceptions of general personality. A five-factor approach to describing basic clusters of personality variables has gained considerable acceptance (e.g., Digman & Inouye, 1986; Goldberg, 1993; McCrae & Costa, 1985). Of the five, two factors are largely interpersonal: extraversion and agreeableness. (See Box 6.2 for a more general discussion of the five-factor model.)

McCrae and Costa (1989), noting the similarity between these two factors and the interpersonal circle dimensions, suggested that the five-factor model provides a framework for the circumplex approach, and the circumplex elaborates on the factors. Trapnell and Wiggins (1990) proposed that the circumplex dimensions of the Interpersonal Adjective Scales (Wiggins, Trapnell, & Phillips, 1988) can serve as markers of the extroversion and agreeableness factors. (They extended those scales to include scales for the remaining three factors of the five-factor model.)

WHAT ARE THE MOST BASIC TRAITS?

Much theorizing and research has been done to characterize human attributes in a comprehensive but succinct format. The goal has been to organize similar attributes into groups so that (1) the number of dispositional clusters is small, giving each broad utility; and (2) most relatively pure attributes are appropriately encompassed in one and only one group. Modern computers and statistical techniques (most notably, factor analysis) allow us to accomplish such grouping in an empirical way. However, we depend on human judgment to decide which factor solution is best. Of particular importance, we must decide how many groups of attributes (each group is called a factor) form the best solution. If too few factors are included, many important attributes will not fit well into any factor; if too many factors are included, the factors become so narrow as to lose broad utility.

A number of studies offer solutions to this problem that are quite similar and strike many researchers as meeting the above goals. These studies propose that five is the best number of broad factors adequately representing the domain of traits. (Not everyone agrees that this is the best solution, however. For example, Eysenck [1992] believes three factors make more sense, and Hogan and Hogan [1992] use six.)

The way in which the five factors are organized sometimes differs a bit across researchers, and a variety of names have been applied to the factors. For example, Costa and McCrae (1993) use the factor labels Extroversion, Agreeableness, Conscientiousness, Neuroticism, and Openness to Experience. Goldberg (1992) organizes the factors somewhat differently, calling them Surgency, Agreeableness, Conscientiousness, Emotional Stability, and Intellect.

BOX 6.2. Five-factor models of personality.

It might also be mentioned that a third factor of this model, adjustment/neuroticism, likely has strong ties to interpersonal functioning. For example, Horowitz and Vitkus (1986) discuss in detail the interplay between relational skill, relationships, and dysfunctional behavior. In the case of the adjustment factor, however, the factor is not itself a collection of interpersonal attributes.

Social Skills

Within psychology, especially from behavioral perspectives, the most common generic label for interpersonal behaviors is social skills. (More recently and in areas other than psychology, such as communication, other terms are more prominent, including social competence and interpersonal competence.) The construct of relational competence is somewhat related to the general rubric of social skill. However, they differ in at least four important ways.

First, social skill often is defined with rather vague boundaries. For example, Phillips (1978, p. 13) views social skills rather broadly as "the extent to which [one] can communicate with others in a manner that fulfills one's rights, requirements, satisfactions, or obligations to a reasonable degree without damaging the other person's similar rights, requirements, satisfactions, or obligations . . . " Libet and Lewinsohn (1973, p. 304) define it in terms of others' response to behavior, "the complex ability both to emit behaviors which are positively or negatively reinforced and not to emit behaviors that are punished or extinguished by others." Bellack and Hersen (1977, p. 145) see it as "an individual's ability to express both positive and negative feelings in the interpersonal context without suffering consequent loss of social reinforcement." In keeping with the concept of relational competence, these writers appear to view social skill as an ability or set of abilities, in part used to manage personal and interpersonal goals. But whereas relational competence focuses on management of relationships themselves, the concept of social skills focuses more on achieving personal goals in social contexts.

Second, in its narrowest form, especially during the early days of social skill intervention, the term came to be almost synonymous with assertiveness. Intervention—social skills training—was often merely assertiveness training.

Third, the social skills approach is strongly associated with behavioral approaches, with its emphasis on situational contingencies. For many it refers most closely to what one does in specific situations, minimizing the emphasis on enduring behavioral tendencies. McFall (1982) criticized two ways the concept of social skills has been used: (1) in reference to stable characteristics of the person, and (2) in a molecular fashion referring to specific component behaviors. He concluded that both approaches were inadequate, proposing instead a two-tiered model that distinguishes between social competence and social skills. Both tiers come from a behavioral perspective. Social competence requires a value judgment concerning effectiveness of performance in a specific task. Social skills are the specific components that may or may not be relevant to performing a task competently. Although such situation-specific analysis of behavior is a valid enterprise, such an approach does not encompass relational competence.

Perhaps most importantly, the concept of social skills has been much more closely tied to molecular social interactions than to relationships. This in part arises from social skill's behavioral emphasis of situational determinants. For example, it is not at all difficult to imagine the psychopath who is socially skilled but relationally incompetent. The psychopath's behavior might be smooth and assertive (i.e., it manages a social exchange well so that immediate goals are realized), but it usually promotes little in terms of closeness and is eventually destructive of relationships.

Masculinity/Femininity

One less obvious but likely related area of study is masculinity/femininity. Research on masculine and feminine roles and the related concept of androgyny has focused on sources, description, and consequences of basic gender differences. However, after examining the nature of gender differences as measured in most studies, Spence (1983) concluded that the two trait clusters actually measured might be better labeled "dominance" and "nurturance/warmth." For example, in his study of relational competence in the elderly, Hansson (1986a) used an adaptation of the Bem Sex Role Inventory, but referred to the dimensions measured as instrumentality and sensitivity. The constructs of masculinity and femininity may well include other features (Spence, 1983), but it does appear that most research on the topic has assessed interpersonal skills which overlap the two-component model of relational competence.

Viewing this research from the perspective of relational skills and relationships has interesting implications. For example most sex-role research has found that androgyny is not superior to masculinity, and that femininity is sometimes associated with emotional vulnerability. Although such findings are troubling if masculinity/femininity are viewed as characterizing the essence of the two sexes, they make sense when viewed from the perspective of relationships. Stereotypes about masculinity/femininity match stereotypes about the relational skills of men versus women—in particular, that women are oriented more toward enhancement. However, enhancement skills demand much of the person but depend on the relational partner for positive outcome. That is, they are *other promoting* rather than *self promoting*. Hence, benefit results indirectly, through stronger relationships.

Stress and Coping

Given the stressful nature of many relationships and the social context of much stress and coping, stress research likely has many implications for relational competence. Carpenter and Scott (1992) outlined reasons for examining stress from the perspective of relationships, including evidence for an interpersonal dimension in stressful situations. From this perspective, relational competence can serve as a coping resource, acting to reduce interpersonal stressors, encourage more positive appraisal, and assist in the development of other resources (such as social support and self-esteem). Hobfoll (1992), recognizing this role of relationships and social functioning, extended this idea to coping. His Strategic Approach to Coping Scale includes subscales for Social Cooperation, Seeking Social Support, and Aggressive–Antisocial Action.

Two particular concepts found in the stress and coping literature are relevant to the construct of relational competence, mastery (e.g., Pearlin & Schooler, 1978) and self-efficacy (Bandura, 1977). Whereas mastery tends to refer to one's sense of global effectiveness, self-efficacy tends to refer more to belief about situation-specific abilities. From this viewpoint, belief in one's relational competence, perhaps as reflected by self-report, is akin to relational self-efficacy or a narrow form of mastery.

MEASUREMENT

It became evident in our early studies that relational competence could not be assessed adequately using existing measures. Most notably, as relational competence became better defined, it became difficult to find measures which, even in combination, sampled well the breadth of the construct. In addition, existing measures varied widely in format, length, reliability, and many existing scales lacked the content specificity that allowed a clean interpretation of findings. Consequently, the Relational Competence Scale (RCS; Carpenter, 1987, 1993a, b) was developed. A self-report approach was selected, although the final instrument readily adapts to permit ratings by others.

Selection of Attributes

As shown earlier in Table 6.2, the range of attributes subsumed under the construct of relational competence is potentially quite broad. The construct was therefore operationalized by sampling from those personal attributes that reflect a skill, are conceptually related to interpersonal dynamics, and have been shown through research to be relevant to the development, use, and maintenance of relationships.

The specific attributes selected for the RCS Initiation component were: assertiveness, dominance, instrumental competence, shyness, and social anxiety (the last two loading negatively). All were judged to be important for developing and accessing relationships in useful ways. The only one not obviously interpersonal, instrumental competence, was included for three primary reasons. Its covariance with relationship measures has been demonstrated in other studies (e.g., Jones et al., 1985), social advantages result from being viewed as capable and skilled, and inclusion of the construct allows closer integration to other, related constructs, such as masculinity.

The specific attributes selected for the Enhancement component include intimacy, trust, interpersonal sensitivity, altruism, and perspective taking. All were judged to be interpersonal in nature and to be skills that can strengthen relationships. Table 6.3 summarizes these constructs and provides examples of items.

Scale Development

Each of the 10 constructs included in the Relational Competence Scale is represented by its own subscale. Subscales were developed using the construct-oriented approach (Wiggins, 1973) and the iterative procedures of Jackson (1970). This simply means that items were written to closely represent a definition of the construct (see examples in Figure 6.3) and repeatedly tried out and rewritten until a group of items remained that worked together to ask about the construct. Based on data from college and noncollege adults, items were selected if they correlated with each other, had lower correlations with other subscales on the RCS, and had low correlations with either social desirability or acquiescence.

The 10 final subscales each include ten items, with balanced keying. Items are answered on a four-point scale, from "strongly agree" to "strongly disagree." Scoring is simply the sum of item weights, with a range from 10 to 40 per subscale. Domain scores for Initiation and Enhancement are the sum of the five relevant subscale scores (after reversing scores for shyness and social anxiety), with a range from 50 to 200.

Scale Attributes

RCS responses have now been collected from over 1,200 subjects, representing normal, clinical, and speciality populations. These data

TABLE 6.3. The Relational Competence Scale

Construct	Description	Sample item
Initiation domain		
Assertiveness	The tendency of the individual to accept, express, actively seek after, and protect reasonable personal needs and desires, including resistance to unreasonable infringements by others	It is sometimes hard for me to stand up for myself when challenged (negatively keyed)
Dominance	The desire and ability to be in charge, at least of one's own situation, and to engage in tasks reflecting leadership, ascendance, and independence	I am a leader in most situations
Instrumental competence	A belief that one is generally capable, skilled, and accomplished, with emphasis on successfully completing tasks or meeting goals	My performance compares very well with that of others
Shyness	The self-perception that one is inhibited and reluctant in social situations, or has poor skill in meeting and getting to know others	Most people say I seem reserved
Social anxiety	Increased feelings of anxiety, worry, and negative self-evaluation in situations involving others, reflecting self-consciousness and especially manifest as the number of others or focus on the subject increases	I am comfortable in a group, even when I am playing a big part (negatively keyed)
Enhancement domain		
Intimacy	The tendency to promote and seek closeness in relationships, especially a few select relationships, by encouraging sharing, deep mutual understanding, mutual interest, and openness	I am able to discuss sensitive experiences with those close to me
Trust	Belief that others are dependable, loyal, and trustworthy, with one's behavior showing such confidence in others	Other people are often undependable when it counts. (negatively keyed)
Interpersonal sensitivity	Attitudes and behavior that show consideration, warmth, and caring and reflect active attempts to be aware of and responsive to others' needs	I usually treat others quite gently

(continued)

TABLE 6.3. (*Continued*)

Construct	Description	Sample item
Altruism	An orientation toward helping and supporting others, especially those in extra need or distress	It seems that I am always helping out others who have problems
Perspective taking	The tendency to view issues from several perspectives, especially that of those with whom one is interacting; the purpose of understanding, appreciating, and showing consideration for others is emphasized	I try to think how others will feel before acting

allow examination of the scale properties and scale validity, as well as the construct validity and utility of relational competence. A few of the psychometric properties of the RCS are presented below, as are a few group differences. The results of several validity studies are described in Chapter 7.

Psychometric Properties

The RCS psychometric properties were consistently strong. There is substantial similarity across scales in difficulty level and variability. Further, frequency distributions and indices of kurtosis and skew suggest that all distributions are approximately normal. Alpha coefficients (an index of how well the items work together) for the ten subscales ranged from .77 to .90. This suggests an adequate level of internal consistency for all subscales, considering their brevity. Alphas for Initiation and Enhancement were .95 and .93, respectively.

A sample of 157 college students completed the RCS twice, with a 14-week interval between testings. Even though the period is relatively long, the test–retest correlations were uniformly high (range of .61 to .84, most in the mid-.70s), suggesting fairly good stability of the constructs measured. Test–retest was .83 for Initiation and .75 for Enhancement. (It may be that Initiation attributes are more stable that those of Enhancement, although differences in measurement adequacy cannot be ruled out at this time.)

Gender Differences

At least some gender differences were expected because of the close similarity between the relational competence constructs and other constructs frequently related to gender roles. Group means and *t* tests for

TABLE 6.4. Gender Comparison of Relational Competence Scales, College and Adult Samples

	College means			Noncollege means		
	Male	Female	*t*	Male	Female	*t*
N	44	79		50	47	
Initiation	150.0	144.9	1.22	143.4	143.7	− 0.08
Assertiveness	30.3	28.2	2.10*	28.6	27.8	0.74
Dominance	29.7	28.4	1.16	29.7	27.7	1.75
Instrumental competence	30.9	30.4	0.48	32.0	30.6	1.54
Shyness (−)	20.9	20.3	0.50	23.2	20.0	2.69**
Social anxiety (−)	20.0	21.8	− 1.77	23.7	22.4	1.11
Enhancement	147.3	151.7	− 1.22	134.6	152.8	− 4.64***
Intimacy	31.9	31.8	0.11	26.2	31.1	− 3.97***
Trust	27.5	28.2	− 0.71	25.0	28.7	− 3.40***
Interpersonal sensitivity	28.3	29.4	− 1.15	26.5	30.0	− 4.13***
Altruism	30.9	32.2	1.66	29.4	32.8	3.89***
Perspective taking	28.7	30.1	− 1.68	27.4	30.2	− 2.98**

$*p < .05, **p < .01, ***p < .001$

two samples are presented in Table 6.4. As can be seen, gender differences primarily occurred for noncollege adults on the enhancement subscales. Even these were rather small. Thus, when these attributes are assessed from the perspective of relational skills rather than sex roles, men and women do not appear to differ that much.

Subscale Intercorrelations

As expected, most subscales within each competence domain were substantially intercorrelated, ranging from .64 to .87. This tells us that initiation attributes tend to go together — assertive individuals tend to also be dominant and outgoing. Similarly, relationship enhancing characteristics are usually found together — trusting individuals are prone to also be sensitive and helpful. Even so, the magnitude of these correlations allows us to conclude that although the five subscales in each domain measure a common underlying variable, each also contributes specific variance. This means that it can still be useful to know about individual characteristics comprising initiation and enhancement — some people may be assertive and dominant in their relationships but still feel shy and socially anxious around strangers, for example.

Our research suggests that the two component scores, Initiation and Enhancement, are slightly correlated ($r = .31$). Thus, initiation and enhancement skills tend to go together only slightly. Although the variance shared by the two components is modest, this is in contrast to Wiggins (1982) and some others who view the two components in their models as orthogonal dimensions. We expect, then, that many people will be either high in both or low in both clusters of skills; fewer people should be high in one cluster and low in the other.

Factor Analysis

From the foregoing, it is evident that initiation skills tend to go together, and that enhancement skills tend to go together, but that the two domains do not overlap much. This is the kind of information that factor analysis is ideally designed to assess. Such analysis helps clarify whether the two-domain model of relational competence is a good one. Because a model already existed, a test was conducted of whether the data fit the model. This test is called *confirmatory factor analysis* because it seeks to confirm the factor model we describe. The data were also analyzed using *exploratory factor analysis,* which does not presuppose a preexisting structure but, instead, seeks to find one that fits the data. Both approaches revealed that our two-component model fits the way people respond to the questions on the RCS. (A more complete and technical description of these analyses can be found in Carpenter, 1993a, b.)

SUMMARY AND CONCLUSIONS

The idea of two global domains of interpersonal skills, each encompassing a variety of specific attributes, appears to have considerable merit. When we consider relationship skills from several perspectives — functions served by relational behaviors, existing ideas about the structure of personality, and the dominant theories of interpersonal functioning — our conclusions converge in a model emphasizing one group of skills for developing relationships and another for maintaining and deepening them.

Structuring interpersonal skills according to *initiation* and *enhancement* domains allows us to organize the wide variety of competencies relevant to successful interpersonal functioning. We are then better able to understand and anticipate the role of these diverse attributes in relationships. Commonalities emerge that might otherwise remain hidden. For example, consider our above argument for appreciating the other-directedness of enhancement as a way of explaining liabilities associated with "femininity," which, from the perspective of sex roles, seem confusing.

Further, as we recognize how one or the other of the two domains is particularly relevant to a relationship challenge, this structure encourages us to consider the variety of attributes subsumed by the domain. By this we mean to remind the reader that specific relational competencies have meaning beyond their inclusion in the domain. For example, it is helpful to first recognize that initiation skills are needed to deal with a particular challenge, but it is also useful to next consider *which* initiation skills. Arriving at the first conclusion naturally leads one to consider the second. Although assertiveness and shyness are conceptually related and have much in common, one's impact on a relationship no doubt differs from the other, depending on the challenge and circumstances. Given the variety and complexity of relationship challenges faced by the elderly (see Tables 5.1 and 5.3), it is likely that the utility of specific competencies will vary within domains. We believe that the ability of the two-component structure to suggest specific attributes provides a powerful tool for understanding relationship successes and failures.

Finally, we have implemented our model into an assessment instrument, the Relational Competence Scale, thereby allowing us to begin testing our ideas. Our initial work is encouraging.

CHAPTER 7

RESEARCH ON RELATIONAL COMPETENCE AND SOCIAL FUNCTIONING

Evidence has now begun to accumulate regarding the impact of relational competence on social functioning and other important outcomes. In this chapter we examine the research pertaining to at least three domains of variables: objective characteristics of relationships (e.g., duration, size, or type of relationship); variables reflecting the quality of one's relationships or interpersonal functioning; and variables previously associated with positive social functioning (e.g., health and well-being). We draw upon our own research in this area and on the numerous studies using individual difference variables subsumed under our comprehensive model of relational competence.

Some of the studies to be described used the Relational Competence Scale (RCS) introduced in Chapter 6. Others relied on alternative measures and approaches to relational competence. Also, much of the initial research has been conducted on younger populations, although many studies involved older adults as well. Conceptually similar research on populations of different ages provides a degree of insight into the continuity of relationships and social interaction across the life-span. It also provides a broader, more basic perspective within which to clarify the role of relational competence in later life.

Our review of the research in this chapter is guided by six basic themes. First, we describe the kind of research we have conducted to assess the validity of the RCS. This helps us develop a psychological profile of those persons who are more (or less) competent and also helps us think about how the construct of relational competence relates to broader theories of personality. A second theme involves the manner in which relational competence impacts social interaction and outcomes resulting from that interaction. A third research question focuses on the relative utility of the Initiation and Enhancement components of relational competence and the situations in which each is most valued. Of particular interest in this connection are those situations involving adaptation to a difficult social transition. A fourth concern is to better understand how the construct of relational competence might fit into broader theories of stress and coping (e.g., in providing coping resources, or altering cognitive stress appraisals). A fifth theme concerns the implications of relational competence for psychological adjustment, well-being, and health. Finally, we review research on relational competence among older adults. Relating back to our model of interpersonal contexts of old age, we propose a research agenda for assessing the role and relevance of interpersonal competencies at each of the suggested stages of dependency and the relational challenges characteristic of that stage.

THE RELATIONAL COMPETENCE SCALE AND MEASURES OF SIMILAR CONSTRUCTS

Because we rely heavily on research conducted with the RCS, it is appropriate to briefly review research on its validity. We examine here three studies. The first compared an individual's self-ratings on the RCS to RCS ratings of the subject by others. This bears on the question of whether self reported relational competence is reflected in observable behavior. The second study compared the RCS to other measures of the attributes sampled by the scale. The third study compared the Initiation and Enhancement domains of the RCS to Leary's Interpersonal Circumplex model and to the constructs of extroversion and agreeableness from the five-factor model of personality (see Chapter 6 for a theoretical discussion of these models and their relationship to relational competence).

Peer Judgments

A sample of 42 married couples and 27 friendship pairs completed the RCS. Each person made two ratings on the RCS; first they described themselves, and then they described their partner. Correlations between self-judgments and judgments by spouse or friend are found in Table 7.1. All correlations were moderately high. We might conclude, then, that not only are most individuals generally aware of their relational competencies, but also that the RCS attributes reflect behavioral distinctions that are observable by others.

TABLE 7.1. Correlations of Relational Competence Subscales with Criterion Measures

	Peer ratings	Criterion measures
N	138	83
Initiation	.55	
Assertiveness	.53	.77
Dominance	.66	.77
Instrumental competence	.55	.68
Shyness (−)	.48	.73
Social anxiety (−)	.44	.81
Enhancement	.49	
Intimacy	.41	
Trust	.46	.46
Interpersonal sensitivity	.52	.78
Altruism	.44	.27
Perspective taking	.30	.68

Note. All correlations but one are significant at $p < .001$. The correlation between altruism and criterion measure is $p < .05$.

Relationships to Measures of Similar Constructs

To establish concurrent validity with previously validated measures, college students completed the RCS, as well as previously established measures of constructs similar to those assessed by the RCS subscales. For example, the Rathus (1973) Assertiveness Schedule was the criterion measure for assertiveness, and the Social Reticence Scale (Jones & Briggs, 1986) was the criterion measure for shyness. No well-validated measure of intimacy, as defined for the RCS, was found (scales of intimacy exist, but these assess the intimacy of a particular dyad rather than the individual's dispositional tendency toward intimacy). Similarly, the measures of trust and altruism used (Wrightsman, 1964) defined the constructs somewhat differently than did the RCS.

Correlations between RCS subscale scores and the designated criterion scales are shown in Table 7.1. They were generally quite large. One exception was altruism, perhaps because the criterion scale was not a good conceptual match. In fact, the correlations between several RCS subscales and their respective criterion scales were nearly as large as the scale reliabilities allowed. Thus, the RCS appears to tap the same constructs as other validated and widely used measures of the target constructs.

The Interpersonal Circumplex, Extroversion, and Agreeableness

The RCS variables were compared to Leary's Interpersonal Circumplex (see Box 6.1 for a review of Leary's model). Because the circumplex is a two-dimensional space we can map RCS variables onto the circumplex. The direction from the circumplex center in which a variable falls reflects the similarity of the variable to the circumplex dimensions, and the distance from the center reflects the strength of the similarity. This mapping (Figure 7.1) reveals that, as expected, both Initiation and Enhancement fall close to the respective circumplex dimensions of dominance–submission (surgency) and love–hate (agreeableness). The fact that they fall near the outer edge of the circumplex indicates that the similarity to these dimensions is strong. Similarly,

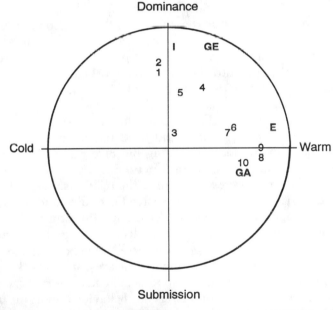

Relational Competence		Goldberg's Adjectives
I = Initiation	E = Enhancement	**GE** = Extroversion
1 = Assertiveness	6 = Intimacy	**GA** = Agreeableness
2 = Dominance	7 = Trust	
3 = Instrumental Competence	8 = Interpersonal Sensitivity	
4 = Shyness (plotted neg.)	9 = Altruism	
5 = Social Anxiety (plotted neg.)	10 = Perspective Taking	

FIGURE 7.1. Relational competence and Leary's Circumplex: Interpersonal circumplex structure of Relational Competence Scales.

when separate RCS subscales were mapped on the circumplex, all except instrumental competence mapped as expected along the two dimensions. Thus, the relational competence model for organizing interpersonal attributes matches reasonably well that proposed earlier by Leary, and available research on the Leary dimensions becomes relevant to our discussion here.

As mentioned in Chapter 6, Trapnell and Wiggins (1990) proposed that Leary's dimensions are nearly identical to two of the "Big Five" dimensions of personality. They renamed those dimensions Surgency and Agreeableness—labels more in keeping with the Big Five literature. Confirmatory factor analysis reveals a good fit for the two-factor model that places Initiation and Wiggins's Surgency in one factor, and Enhancement and Wiggins's Agreeableness in the other. Some other theorists tend to emphasize dimensions slightly different from that of Wiggins. For example, Goldberg (1992) proposes dimensions of Extroversion (rather than Surgency) and Agreeableness. Goldberg's measure also provides a good match to the relational competence domains of Initiation and Enhancement, although the match is not as close as with Wiggins's measure. For comparison, Goldberg's dimensions are also mapped onto the circumplex in Figure 7.1. Similarly, in our research we find Costa and McCrae's (1985, 1993) NEO Extroversion and Agreeableness to correlate highly with Initiation and Enhancement, respectively. These established similarities between our relational competence constructs and these five-factor constructs allow us to apply the rapidly expanding Big Five personality research to relationships and interpersonal functioning.

As an aside, it is interesting to note the relationship of relational competence variables to the other three five-factor dimensions, as measured by Costa and McCrae's NEO Personality Inventory (1985). We find essentially no relationship between RCS scales and Openness to Experience. However, modest positive correlations exist between Conscientiousness and RCS Enhancement measures. It seems that Conscientiousness, including its attention to detail and conformity to social expectations, is relevant to other-serving behavior important in Enhancement. In contrast, we find substantial correlations between Neuroticism and nearly all RCS subscales, even though RCS scales are careful to avoid inquiring about negative mood, personal distress, and other characteristics relevant to the construct of neuroticism. Although these correlations do not confirm cause, it is not surprising that distressed, dysfunctional individuals report impaired relationships and social functioning; neurotic attributes likely contribute to poor social behaviors and visa versa.

PERSONALITY VERSUS BEHAVIOR

The association of traditional personality characteristics with overt behaviors has been the focus of much discussion (e.g., Epstein, 1980; Mischel, 1973). Arguments range from two extremes: (1) only what one does actually counts, and grouping behaviors into supposedly stable tendencies is illusory and without predictive validity; versus (2) a focus on behaviors analyzes human interaction at too microscopic a level to have utility, and the study of traits is a valid and validated enterprise. This discussion is relevant to relational competence. Do the somewhat global characteristics that we emphasize in relational competence, usually assessed by self-report, have anything to do with one's actual behavior? If they did not, the impact of relational competence, as we have described it, would be limited to the individual (and, perhaps, mostly to the way one thinks about relationships). There would be little impact on actual social functioning because a social unit is involved. However, we believe the evidence regarding personality supports three conclusions:

1. Whereas traits are not particularly good for predicting specific behaviors, many are reasonably good at predicting typical behaviors (behavioral tendencies). In fact, attempts to predict specific behaviors are mostly futile, whereas behavioral tendencies—specifically because of their generality—are more likely to tell us important things about people.
2. The association between traits and behavior varies as a function of the trait under consideration. That is, some traits are strongly related to behavior, whereas others are not. Thus, the behavioral consequences of specific traits must be established.
3. The best prediction of behavior probably comes from consideration of both personality and environmental factors. The interaction between traits and situations is, therefore, an important area of study.

BOX 7.1. The relationship between traits and behavior.

SOCIAL INTERACTION AND RELATIONSHIPS

As expected, relational competence attributes reliably predict a person's performance in a wide variety of social interactions. Typically, greater competence is correlated with higher levels of social interaction and better outcomes within that interaction.

Shyness

The research on shyness provides an excellent example of how poor relational competencies can impact social interaction and relationships. Shy, socially anxious individuals tend to date less (Curran, 1977), prefer to work alone rather than with others (McGovern, 1976), participate less in social activities (Jones & Russell, 1982), and conform in ways that minimize drawing attention to themselves (Santee & Maslach, 1982). Such social avoidance is not surprising, given the finding that shy individuals tend to experience discomfort and inhibition in the presence of others (e.g., Cheek & Buss, 1981).

Closer examination suggests rather specific ways in which shyness contributes to difficulties in social interactions. In particular, shy individuals tend to behave in ways that reduce their social potency. Shy students tend to sit near the back and sides of the classroom, where they may remain withdrawn when uncertain and participate only when they feel more competent (Dykman & Reis, 1979). They speak less, tend not to interrupt, contribute disproportionately to a lack of fluency in conversation (e.g., long, uncomfortable pauses), and are slower in responding to conversational partners (e.g., Natale, Entin, & Jaffe, 1979). In interacting with women, men's shyness strongly impacts both their verbal and nonverbal behavior. Shy men speak less and for shorter periods, convey less positive affect, and engage in less eye contact (Garcia, Stinson, Ickes, Bissonnette, & Briggs, 1991). Studies suggest that shyness is readily observed by others (Funder & Dobroth, 1987), so these behaviors are likely to impact social encounters.

In a series of studies (e.g., Hansson, 1986b) we have found that these characteristics and consequences of shyness extend to older populations as well. Further, special social situations common to elderly persons — such as life disruption following loss of a spouse or need for help due to declining abilities — are also negatively impacted by shyness. For example, we find that shy persons have greater fear of crime, viewing their neighborhoods as more hostile and helping resources as less accessible (Hansson & Carpenter, 1986).

Interestingly, the social deficits of shy persons are similar to those found in lonely individuals. For example, when conversing with strangers, lonely individuals are less likely to refer to the conversational partner, continue a topic initiated by the partner, or ask questions (Jones, Hobbs, & Hockenbury, 1982). It is interesting also that college students who are lonely at the beginning of their freshmen year tend to remain lonely if they judge their loneliness to be their own fault and the result of their own poor social behavior. In contrast, students who attribute their loneliness to just leaving home and the newness of school are likely to overcome their initial loneliness (Cutrona, 1982). Persons in the latter group apparently see themselves as socially capable, and they proceed with the task of developing a new social group.

We have extended these findings for lonely individuals to older groups (Hansson, Jones, Carpenter, & Remondet, 1986). As with younger persons, lonely older adults were dissatisfied with their relationships and less well adjusted. In addition, lonely older widows were less likely to have sought out similar others with whom to compare notes (or feelings) regarding the experience of becoming widowed. They were also less likely to have engaged in rehearsals of those behaviors, skills, and consequences that might prove useful in their impending widowhood (such as making new friends). Loneliness among older persons was also associated with perceptions that their community was less predictable or safe. Lonely older persons had less knowledge about available community services for older adults and more negative attitudes toward people who use such services. As a further tie-in to relational competence, we found that loneliness in this older sample was correlated with shyness, external locus of control, and lack of assertiveness.

The more global consequences of shy, lonely persons' deficient social behaviors can be substantial. Researchers find that shy persons are not only rated as more shy by observers, but also as less assertive and friendly (Pilkonis, 1977) and lower in poise and talent (Jones, Cavert, & Indart, 1983). The negative reactions cut both ways, in that after a social exchange shy persons are inclined to rate their partners as less friendly (Jones & Briggs, 1984). Jones and Carpenter (1986) found strong correlations between shyness and loneliness, concluding that shy persons are dissatisfied with their relationships, seeing them as failing to meet their needs. They also found that shy persons report fewer friends, less closeness with friends, and less social support, underscoring the impact of shyness on the whole relational structure of shy individuals.

Initiation Skills and Social Transition

Shyness is a particularly well researched social attribute, but other initiation skills have also received attention. For example, Watson, Clark, McIntyre, and Hamaker (1992) found that persons high in extraversion engage in more socializing. Similarly, extraversion was positively related to longitudinally measured adjustment to aging among men (Costa, McCrae, & Norris, 1981). Hansson, Slade, Nelson, Carpenter, and Rountree (1983) found that assertive senior adults had more contact with others and were more satisfied with their relationships.

Using the Relational Competence Scale, Carpenter (1993b) found Initiation skills to be associated with a variety of positive social outcomes. Initiators (assertive, outgoing people) were less lonely and less anxious. They reported more friendships, more closeness in their friendships, and more social support. The Initiation component of relational competence appeared especially important for those individuals in social transition (such as starting college or moving to a new city).

Shaver, Furman, and Buhrmester (1985) also studied the impact of various social skills on students in their first year at college. They found that social skills (including self-disclosure and assertiveness) were useful for predicting satisfaction with relationships. Skill at meeting new people (which they called initiation skill) was particularly helpful in the fall, just after students left home and old friendships behind. Skilled students were less lonely and more likely to take charge of their social lives by engaging in positive social activities. Interestingly, these skills were less predictive of relationship satisfaction as the school year wore on; apparently, the social transition to college made such skills especially relevant early on when transition was greatest.

In a study of midlevel managers recently transferred by their employers, we found an interesting twist to the usual finding that social competence is especially relevant at times of social transition (Carpenter, 1993b). Life satisfaction among these relocated managers was not particularly dependent on their relational competence. Even those low on initiation skills reported satisfactory social involvement. The built-in social climate of the new work situation appeared to provide a new social network for these relocated workers—thus, they weren't dependent on their own skill for developing new relationships. However, life satisfaction among these recent arrivals was highly dependent on their spouses' satisfaction, and their spouses' satisfaction was partly a function of the spouses' relational competence and involvement in new relationships. Spouses who were shy, unassertive, or socially anxious were simply not making new friends. Thus, it seems that at times of life transition, if social structure is low and opportunities for interaction do not automatically result from situational factors, we are more dependent on our social competencies for relationship development.

Social competencies also appear to influence the way in which we anticipate social transition. For example, among the elderly, shy persons report greater disruption in their lives following major life events of later life, such as retirement, widowhood, and change of residence (Hansson, 1986a). Fletcher and Hansson (1991) studied the role of individual differences in older workers nearing retirement age. They found that shy, lonely workers reported greater retirement anxiety, whereas those high in control both in masculinity (instrumental competence) and femininity (interpersonal sensitivity) experienced less anxiety. The more competent individuals apparently anticipated an easier transition. That is, they expected less difficulty in making new friends, staying socially involved, avoiding loneliness, and so forth. However, more recent work (e.g., Morrison & Hansson, 1993) suggests some refinement to these conclusions. The relationship between social competence and retirement anxiety may be moderated by how close one is to retirement. Older workers who were not that close to retirement (ages 50–55) experienced less anxiety if they were high on enhancement characteristics; initiation was unrelated to anxiety. In contrast, those closest to retirement (over age 55) experienced less anxiety if they were high in initiation skills; enhancement no longer correlated with retirement anxiety. It seems that workers good at promoting current relationships feel secure when retirement is still far off, but as retirement looms closer, the ability to develop new relationships leads to feelings of security.

Enhancement

A number of writers (e.g., Duck, 1988b) have suggested that intimacy-promoting behaviors are particularly relevant to developing and maintaining relationships. Unfortunately, much of the research in this area focuses exclusively on what people do in particular relationships. Less attention has been paid to the broader theoretical question of how enduring attributes such as personality contribute to these relationship-enhancing behaviors. Much work remains to be done, therefore, to clarify how the Enhancement component of relational competence contributes to the task of keeping and improving relationships. However, a number of studies suggest this is a potentially fruitful area.

For example, Gurtman (1992) found that lack of trust was associated with a variety of interpersonal difficulties, including lowered sociability, lack of submissiveness, low intimacy, and a tendency to be too controlling. In contrast, Carlo and his associates (Carlo, Eisenberg, Troyer, Switzer, & Speer, 1991) found that those high in trait altruism were likely to volunteer to help distressed others, even though the persons to be helped were strangers and helping required personal expense.

Jones and Vaughan (1990) found communal orientation (being oriented toward the needs and concerns of the partner) enhanced satisfaction of best friendships among older adults. Similarly, higher communal orientation was associated with less depression among caregivers of Alzheimer patients (Williamson & Schulz, 1990).

Davis and Carpenter (1987) found marital satisfaction to be much higher among persons whose spouses were seen as high in Enhancement, including the attributes of intimacy, trust, interpersonal sensitivity, altruism, and perspective taking. Interestingly, one's own Enhancement did not correlate very highly with one's marital satisfaction—people want enhancing spouses but don't necessarily benefit from being enhancing themselves.

Yeatts (1993), in a study of problems with mentoring relationships in the workplace, found an interesting role for relational competence of those being mentored. Specifically, persons high in Enhancement were much less likely to expect problems to arise in the mentoring relationship (e.g., exploitation, betrayal, or neglect). Initiation made no difference. Workers with high enhancement skills expected that their ability to work out problems and foster the positive side of relationships would serve them well in their relationship with mentors.

Under some circumstances, however, enhancement behaviors may contribute to relationship problems. Carpenter (1993a) suggested that enhancement skills, because they most directly benefit others, depend on a positive relationship for the enhancing individual to experience positive outcomes. If one offers kindness, intimacy, and trust to an angry, unaccepting partner, vulnerability to hurt is greatly increased. A study of distressed couples' marital communication by Sayers and Baucom (1991) yielded such results. These researchers found that femininity (i.e., interpersonal sensitivity and tendency to express emotion) was associated with a tendency for wives to engage in more and longer negative interactions, and to reciprocate husbands' negative communication. Within a hostile relationship, it seems that efforts to focus on feelings only tended to prolong and accentuate a couple's negative exchanges.

RELATIONAL COMPETENCE AND SUCCESSFUL AGING

In Chapter 2 we introduced the concept of successful aging and argued that society must learn from those older individuals who have not followed the "usual" trajectory of age-related declines in the functional areas of their lives. In this context, we have begun to study successful aging in the workplace. Perry and Hansson (1992) conducted interviews of highly successful older men and women in large work organizations and identified personal characteristics that contributed to successful aging within work organizations. Four important characteristics emerged to highlight the value of social competence. First, these individuals were high in sociability. They were outgoing, liked social involvement, and were inclined to see social exchanges as important vehicles for job success. Second, they treated others with courtesy and respect. In particular, they did not appear manipulative in this regard; in contrast, this was their manner with everyone, regardless of status. Third, they maintained good emotional control. Although not strictly social, this skill was important for positively impacting others, perhaps by instilling trust. Fourth, they attracted both influential mentors and faithful followers. This led to training and experiences that helped their careers, as well as a network of supportive others within the organization.

Perry and Hansson (1991) also studied a sample of older workers to determine the impact of relational skill on one's ability to retain organizational power and influence until late in one's work life. They found that older employees high in initiation skills were most likely to report having retained their power and influence in the workplace. Not surprisingly, enhancement skills were unrelated to having power and influence. Similarly, in a study of age-related risks during job change, Bailey and Hansson (1993) found that concern over these risks was associated with initiation, such that greater concern was expressed by persons high in shyness and external locus of control and low in instrumental competence.

We noted in early chapters that evaluations of an elderly person's ability to live independently often include an assessment of social capacity. Not only have interpersonal factors become a part of formal assessments, but their importance also appears to be broadly understood by the families of frail, elderly persons and by older persons themselves. For example, among nonshy older individuals, attitudes toward one's own aging are largely a function of one's health and independence; in contrast, among shy older persons, attitudes reflect more one's social abilities, network size, and interaction with family (Hansson, 1986b). Hansson, Nelson, et al. (1990) studied the factors that influence family members when they consider intervening in the decisions or independent living arrangements of an elderly parent. As might be expected, health and physical limitations were prominently mentioned. However, social stressors—such as widowhood, retirement, and loss of social network—were also major factors in families' evaluations. These researchers also found that family consciousness about aging issues and level of family involvement in caregiving for the older parent tended to be higher if the parent was unmarried, alone, shy, and low in masculinity. It appears that families recognize the social vulnerability of the older family member and attempt to compensate.

STRESS AND COPING

Stress and coping theory suggests that people with more coping resources should experience less stress when demands are heavy and be more effective in dealing with those demands. Three general predictions can be made regarding those with greater relational competence:

- Their relationship resources will be high; additional resources will positively impact the stress process.
- They will experience less stress from social stressors because their better social functioning results in fewer stressors and because stressors that do occur are less threatening.
- Their preference will be greater for coping strategies that are social in nature, and they will be more effective in drawing on social coping resources.

Our own work and that of others suggests that all three predictions are accurate (although the third hypothesis has been less extensively studied). For example, as noted above, those high in relational competence report more friends, higher social support, and greater satisfaction with relationships. In turn, a huge literature points to (at least moderate) benefits of social support in reducing stress and associated problems (cf. Sarason, Sarason, & Pierce, 1990).

A number of individual difference variables have become prominent in the stress and coping literature, particularly as personal coping resources. For example, Pearlin and Schooler (1978) demonstrated that mastery and self-esteem are reliable predictors of stress outcomes. Such persons have a general sense of competence that appears to buffer the negative effects of stress. Neither mastery nor self-esteem are necessarily social in nature. However, we believe self-concept is heavily influenced by social functioning, and we find both variables to be highly correlated with our construct of relational competence. Similarly, Bandura (1977) proposed the construct of self-efficacy, a belief in one's ability to perform particular tasks. This too has been shown to be related to coping and stress outcomes. Relational competence, from this perspective, is a somewhat generalized form of relational self-efficacy.

Finally, locus of control is a factor in the stress process, with those having an internal locus of control (a tendency to take control or see themselves as having control) experiencing better stress outcomes. Locus of control appears to be a multifaceted construct (e.g., Lefcourt, 1991), in which one component is clearly social, sharing much with variables falling within the initiation domain of relational competence, such as assertiveness and dominance.

We see, then, that relational competence is clearly associated with having relationship resources likely to benefit the individual experiencing stress. Further, personal characteristics found to be important in the stress process are closely allied to relational competence. The remainder of this section presents findings supporting our second and third hypotheses.

Social Stressors

Rook (1984) studied the negative side of social interaction among elderly women. She found that 38% of those who created problematic situations for her participants were friends, and another 36% were family. She also found that negative social relationships had more impact on well-being than did positive relationships. This should not be surprising. Not only are many of the very people on whom one relies for support likely to be a major source of stress, but because such relationships are ongoing, the potential for continued stress is high. (The reader will recall we discussed this issue in some detail in Chapters 3 and 4.)

To clarify the role of social functioning in stress, Carpenter and Scott (1990) had people rate the similarity of different kinds of stressors, from major traumatic events such as the death of a spouse to minor but frequent troubles such as managing finances. Participants were not informed that the focus of the study was actually to evaluate the relational component of stress; they were asked only to judge overall similarity of each stressor to every other stressor. Empirical techniques for clarifying what dimensions underlie these judgments revealed that the interpersonal nature of stressors was particularly important. That is, regardless of other similarities and differences, judges tended to see two stressors as alike if they were interpersonal in nature but different if one was interpersonal and the other was not.

If the social aspect of stressors is important, it is likely that social competence assists people as they cope with such stressors. In fact, we find that those high in relational competence report less relational stress. They even report less stress overall, whether focusing on the subjective feeling of being stressed or listing the particular demands on them. This finding is strongest when the type of social competence studied is of the initiation type and when the stressors are social. Under such circumstances, for example, shy individuals describe themselves as more stressed and, in particular, report more relational stress (Carpenter, 1985).

Appraisal of Social Stressors

Cognitive models of stress emphasize an evaluative component in the stress process called appraisal (Lazarus & Folkman, 1984). When some demand is placed upon us we evaluate its potential impact and our capacity to deal with it. Under the cognitive model, if our appraisal leads us to believe we will be overwhelmed, we react with a stress response of anxiety, worry, depression, or the like.

In a recent study, Carpenter and Suhr (1988) examined the relationship between threat appraisal and relational competence. Participants were given a stressful task of a social nature and, prior to beginning the task, asked to appraise three aspects of the task: (1) recognition that the task is demanding; (2) caring about the task because it leads to important consequences; and (3) beliefs that one has resources to cope with the demand and that one will succeed. They then completed the task and completed measures of how they felt during the task. As expected, all three forms of appraisal were highly correlated with stressful emotions during and after the task. Those who appraised the task as demanding or important or who appraised themselves as unskilled or unlikely to succeed tended to experience more worry, fear, tension, passivity, and embarrassment. The finding of most interest here, however, was that scores on the RCS also predicted the nature of the stress appraisal. Those high on Initiation rated their resources and likelihood of success more positively and the task as less difficult. High scorers on Enhancement had a similar pattern. Interestingly, Initiation but not Enhancement was also correlated with appraisal of task importance, such that high initiators saw their performance as less important and less relevant to their self-image.

These results, then, suggest a number of ways in which relational competence can be quite relevant to stress appraisal. However, some of our more recent work suggests that this may partly depend on the nature of the stressor. As we have emphasized throughout this book, relational skills ought to be most helpful for dealing with social challenges. In the above study the demand to be appraised was social, whereas in our more recent work, participants appraised and experienced a nonsocial stressor. For this latter group, relational competence still significantly predicted appraisal, but the prediction was not as strong. The results suggest that those high in relational competence still saw themselves as capable individuals, but they probably placed greater emphasis on attributes relevant to the task at hand for making their appraisals.

Social Coping

One need not deal with exclusively social stressors to benefit from relationships and relational skills. For example, Hansson, Briggs, et al. (1990) studied the connections between social competence and emotional outcomes in chronically unemployed older persons. They found, as do others, that chronically unemployed persons commonly experience depression, loneliness, and a sense of lowered personal control. However, shyness, perspective taking, and assertiveness—all components of relational competence—were also strong predictors of these negative outcomes. In fact, social abilities reliably predicted loneliness and perceived control even after unemployment factors were taken into account. Contrary to popular conceptions, the emotional reactions of these older persons seemed to be largely due to their social functioning and not just to their difficulties in finding work.

ADJUSTMENT AND WELL-BEING

Much of the evidence we have already presented reveals that those with higher relational competence accept challenges with less distress, are more confident of their abilities, and engage in behaviors that are functional. In addition, we find strong ties between relational competence and well-being variables. For example, we, along with others, find that the initiation component of relational competence is highly correlated with self-esteem. We find this with college students (Jones et al., 1985), medical patients (Carpenter et al., 1983), widows, and older persons in general (Hansson, 1986b). Interestingly, although enhancement characteristics positively impact relationships, they are not particularly good predictors of well-being.

We find that relational competence is also a good predictor of specific attitudes and emotional states as well. For example, older persons generally report greater fear of crime. However, this association is particularly strong among the shy elderly, who seem to find their social surroundings less supportive and focus more on potential threats (Hansson, 1986b).

As mentioned earlier in this chapter, relational competence is also associated with neuroticism, which reflects emotional and behavioral adjustment. Both initiation and enhancement competencies are associat-

---

A PARADOX WITH SOCIAL SUPPORT

We, along with others, have found an interesting twist to the usual result that more socially competent individuals are more effective at using social ways of coping. This finding is that those who report greater social support (they think more people are supportive of them, and they are more satisfied with the support they feel) also report lower reliance on others to help solve their problems. These people are, in effect, saying that support is available but they are disinclined to use it when difficulties arise. Further, it is sometimes found that those who are high users of social support have lower self-esteem and poorer scores on other indicators of well-being.

Relational competence helps make sense of this seeming paradox. Social support is correlated with both Initiation and Enhancement, but more strongly with Initiation. Not surprisingly, those who make friends easily and relate readily to others report many supportive others; these people tend to have good self-esteem and social confidence, and hence, are inclined to be positive about how others like them. However, Initiation, including constructs like dominance, assertiveness, and self-confidence, is also correlated with measures of independence, mastery, and control. Those high in Initiation are inclined to choose to maintain independence and control; their esteem comes in part from their ability to take care of themselves.

Indeed, if people turn too readily to others for help (especially when problems are of the sort they believe they should be able to handle alone) it is hard to take credit for a success. Such persons might instead feel incompetent or dependent. Thus, the support helps deal with the stressor but lowers self-image. Further, such dependency may interfere with relationships, making the dependent person feel more vulnerable. Successful users of supportive others, then, are probably careful not to overdo it.

BOX 7.2. Feeling supported versus using support.

ed with lower neuroticism. Relational competence is also correlated with more extreme forms of maladjustment, as found in psychiatric patients. For example, alcoholics and psychiatric patients score lower on the Relational Competence Scale that do normal subjects. Psychiatric patients are much lower than normals on Initiation attributes, with alcoholics falling in between. For Enhancement, the pattern is reversed (Carpenter, 1993a). These findings are consistent with theories about social functioning within alcoholism, in which disruption of close relationships and the manipulation of others is prominent. In contrast, psychiatric patients seem most deficient in the more public behaviors of Initiation. Psychiatric patients also score poorly on closeness promoting Enhancement behaviors such as Intimacy and Trust, with nearly normal scores on Enhancement behaviors reflecting consideration of others, such as interpersonal sensitivity and perspective taking.

HEALTH

There is relatively little work specifically relating relational competence to health. However, allied lines of research suggest this would be a fruitful area. For example, the ties between social support and health, although often of modest size, are well established and diverse (Cohen & Syme, 1985). For example, lowered support is associated with increased risk for mortality (Berkman, 1985), cardiovascular disease (Welin et al., 1985), and survival among cancer patients (Reynolds & Kaplan, 1990). The importance of social support as a risk factor in cardiovascular disease is roughly equivalent to other known risk factors, such as smoking and high cholesterol (Atkins et al., 1991). Given the substantial role of relational competence in the development of social support, indirect ties between social competence and health are likely.

An interesting example of the intertwined nature of social competence and social support together impacting health behavior is shown in the reactions of older persons to impairment of their abilities to perform the activities of daily living. Such impairment is a natural outcome of declines in health and sensory capacity. Hansson (1986b) found that for nonshy individuals such impairment was correlated with poorer health, spending more time alone, and feeling more vulnerable. But these nonshy persons also accommodated reality, seeking and accepting support from others to balance their declines. In contrast, shy older persons' impairment in daily living activities was not associated with health, time alone, and vulnerability. Instead, it seemed that shy persons felt alone and vulnerable regardless of their impairment in daily living activities. In particular, shy persons were likely to let social barriers (such as embarrassment or fear of strangers) keep them from needed help and social services, a tendency that put the impaired among them at higher risk (Hansson, 1986b).

There have been numerous efforts to relate stable individual differences to specific illnesses, mostly without success. However, most earlier attempts looked for a single type of individual prone to the illness in question, ignoring the likelihood that multiple characteristics are at work. They tended to emphasize older concepts of personality, especially from the psychoanalytic tradition of internal conflicts, and they did not integrate personality and social functioning with other risk factors. In spite of limitations, a few approaches have been successful. For example, Kobasa (1979) characterized a group of people with good health, even in the face of stress. These "hardy" individuals differed from less healthy persons in that they were more *committed* to major areas of their as family and work, believed they were in *control* of major life influences, and viewed life demands as *challenges* rather than threats.

Type A

Perhaps the most notable line of research contrasting person characteristics of healthy versus nonhealthy individuals is that of the Type A pattern. Friedman and Rosenman (1974) described Type A individuals as impatient, competitive and achievement oriented to the point of aggressiveness, and prone to anger when provoked or when goals are blocked. These people are typically energetic and are often heavily committed to work. A number of major studies reveal that these fast-paced individuals are substantially more vulnerable to heart disease (Friedman & Booth-Kewley, 1987).

However, over time it has become increasingly clear that many of the features of the Type A personality as originally described are not related to illness-proneness. Being energetic and emotionally expressive seem unimportant to the development of heart disease, as do time urgency and job involvement. Rather, hostility and anger stand out as the most relevant characteristics (Smith, 1992). Those who seem to demand control over their situations, have a need to dominate others, and respond aggressively to others when their control is threatened are the ones who have increased risk for heart disease.

Although not exclusively social, the interpersonal nature of hostility and anger are significant. A number of writers have particularly noted that hostility seems to occur when high competitiveness exists in conjunction with mistrust, suspicion, and self-interest at the expense of others (e.g., Barefoot et al., 1987). The interpersonal components, in relational competence terms, might be comparable to high dominance and assertiveness combined with low caring and trust. Hansson et al. (1983) also noted a similar combination of interpersonal factors in the Type A construct. They suggested it included a combination of career-involvement factors (such as ambition) and self-defeating interpersonal behaviors (such as low empathy and low interpersonal perceptiveness).

A variety of hypotheses exist regarding how these characteristics, some of them quite social, affect health. For example, Kaplan et al. (1993) suggested that hostile people (Type As) appear to experience more interpersonal conflict and may respond more dramatically to social stressors. This exaggerated physiological responding could be the source of cardiovascular damage.

Alcoholism

A variety of behavioral and psychological disorders have implications for health. Particularly notable among them is alcoholism, frequently damaging important body systems such as the liver or nervous system, often leading to poor health habits, and contributing to bodily injury through accidents (e.g., DiMatteo, 1991). The suspected causes of alcoholism are varied and complex, including genetics, physical reactions to alcohol, and psychological mechanisms. Social factors no doubt play an important role in the development of alcoholism and in resistance to treatment. For example, the social context of drinking is prominent in our society and is often given as a reason for differing alcoholism rates across cultures.

Several studies have found that a few personality patterns are particularly common among alcoholics (e.g., Graham & Strenger, 1988). For example, one pattern characterizes individuals as prone to reject societal norms, typically scoring high on measures of hostility and lack of constraint; another pattern is of the anxious, socially withdrawn individual who learns that alcohol blunts the negative feelings brought on by stress and poor social interaction. Again, social competencies appear relevant to these vulnerable individuals. With the development of clearer ties between individual differences and social functioning that are now emerging, we will hopefully see more clearly how personality and relationships contribute to this and other health-threatening disorders.

Health Behaviors in Old Age

In old age, health problems typically increase and are often more difficult to diagnose and treat. Thus, healthy behaviors—as well as other behaviors that promote effective treatment when illness does occur—are particularly important.

The doctor–patient relationship is often critical to good health care and, as a relationship, is dependent on the interpersonal skills of both physician and patient. For example, Hansson et al. (1988) noted that negative experiences with a physician are common, frequently resulting in failure to return to that doctor. They found that most reasons given for changing doctors involved poor interpersonal behavior by the physician (e.g., not listening, showing disinterest, or acting condescendingly) rather than concerns over technical competence.

A number of researchers have noted the limited dialogue that occurs between doctors and their patients, perhaps in part because of the increasing dominance of technology in modern medicine (see Chapter 3 for related discussion of this topic). For example, Waitzkin and Stoeckle (1976) found that during medical visits, typically lasting 20 minutes, doctors averaged less than 1 minute of giving information to the patient. In contrast, the doctors thought they were spending 50% to 75% of this time communicating. Also, physicians are often ineffective in their instructions to patients, frequently giving or changing prescriptions without explaining them to the patient, and rarely writing down information or checking to see if instructions are understood. Similarly, patients rarely ask questions and rapidly forget much of what the physician tells them. A common complaint is that doctors don't listen to what they say, but few patients correct apparent misunderstandings in the information they give or tell the doctor when they don't understand something. Elderly persons seem particularly reluctant to play an assertive role in the medical consultation, perhaps because of older norms about the dominant status of the doctor. Further, vague, multiple complaints of illness common to older persons make effective communication especially critical. It is evident, then, that the relational skills of both doctor and patient are important to effective treatment. But whereas much recent work has highlighted the importance of productive social interaction, very little has explored how social competencies aid this kind of social transaction.

Relational competencies have also been linked to health behaviors in other ways. For example, in a study of three groups of vulnerable adults (permanently disabled para/quadraplegics, diabetics, and older adults), we studied the relationship of assertiveness to health practices and adjustment to medical conditions (Hansson, Slade, Nelson, Carpenter, & Rountree, 1983). We found that assertive individuals were better adjusted emotionally, less physically dependent, more compliant with prescribed treatment regimens, and more satisfied with relationships.

CONCLUSIONS

Our review of relational competence research reveals strong ties between competence, social functioning, and a number of important outcomes. Particularly well established is the positive impact of relational competence on (1) friendships among relatively autonomous individuals, (2) social transitions common to older and younger adults, such as moving to new neighborhoods, and (3) effectively coping with stressful events. This body of research is quite supportive of the conclusion that social competence and effective relationships enhance life functioning generally and are relevant to many challenges faced by elders specifically.

However, as we compare this work to our earlier outline of relational challenges (Tables 5.1 and 5.3), we find that most research focuses on concerns that impact all age groups, such as making new friends. The role of relational competence remains unexplored for a number of challenge domains. This is particularly true as we move toward the challenges associated with greater dependency (e.g., the relational skills relevant to successful entry into an institution). Admittedly, greater dependency is related to more severe health problems and physical limitations, greater involvement from professionals, and institutional settings. As the importance of these other factors grows, it is likely that the capacity of relational competence to make a difference is diminished (as suggested by Figure 5.1). Even so, we anticipate that prior to extreme feebleness and dependency, the usefulness of relational competencies can be substantial, augmenting the benefits of good care.

We also note an interesting trend in the study of relational functioning with increasing dependency. For relatively autonomous elders, the focus is most often directly on the older adult. But as dependency increases, research shifts toward studying the caregiver. No doubt, the contribution of the caregiver extends beyond physical care into relationship, particularly when we note most caregivers are family members. (See Chapter 9 for a discussion of relational functioning and caregivers.)

Many questions still remain. We hope to see at least four general trends in future research: (1) relating relational functioning of the older adult to the challenges most unique to aging and dependency, such as adjustment to institutional care; (2) development and evaluation of new intervention programs for relational competencies—especially enhancement skills—as is now done with assertiveness; (3) learning what factors lead to the strong family and friendship ties that do last through periods of dependency; and (4) longitudinal research to characterize how enduring socially relevant dispositions impact relationships and well-being as age-related challenges evolve.

CHAPTER 8

INTERVENTION STRATEGIES

The growing elderly population and an increasing awareness of this group's needs are resulting in a proliferation of treatments targeted for older clients. Many of these treatments focus on the older person's social functioning or have implications for that functioning. They are the primary focus of this chapter. In spite of its breadth and importance, however, only a modest amount of research has critically examined interventions designed specifically for older adults (Smyer, Zarit, & Qualls, 1990). Such a mismatch between treatment implementation and evaluation is typical for a population of emerging interest, but it undermines our ability to draw conclusions about the efficacy or mechanisms of many treatments. It will be important in the near future to conduct the intervention research that will permit treatment decisions for older adults to be made largely on the basis of empirical studies.

A number of general treatment issues are briefly discussed in this chapter. However, those interested in broader examinations are referred to other collections. For example, readers interested in treatment accessibility and therapist attitudes toward the elderly are referred to Gatz, Popkin, Pino, and VandenBos (1985) or to Smyer et al. (1990). Those interested in intervention generally might consult one of several good handbooks, such as the *Handbook of Psychotherapy and Behavior Change* (Garfield & Bergin, 1987).

The remainder of the chapter explores issues that arise in the treatment of older persons (especially when interpersonal functioning seems to be a contributing factor to the individual's problem). In this context, we provide a model for conceptualizing the range of interventions that might enhance interpersonal functioning and its benefits. We discuss the nature of relational stress and why the functions of assessment, problem identification, goal setting, and treatment planning become more complex when dealing with older persons. Finally, we review examples of traditional treatment approaches that have (with some success) been adapted for use with older adults.

GENERAL ISSUES

Four main considerations seem particularly relevant in the treatment of older persons. First, it is frequently unclear which features of geriatric treatments make them unique, as compared to traditional treatment of younger adults. The intervention literature often fails to distinguish between age groups, with most studies that are relevant to older persons freely intermingling older and younger clients. We find this neither surprising nor inappropriate, since most therapeutic processes for older persons seem similar to those of younger persons (cf. Gatz et al., 1985). When age-group differences do emerge, they are often modest, and treatment considerations for a large proportion of elderly clients will not differ from younger clients. In fact, studies suggest that most older persons respond well to traditional treatment (e.g., Gatz, 1988; Horowitz, Marmar, Weiss, DeWitt, & Rosenbaum, 1984; Pinkston & Linsk, 1984; Thompson, Gallagher, & Breckenridge, 1987). Moreover, age-related assumptions on the part of therapists—especially those regarding limited treatment efficacy with older clients—are often inappropriate and can lead to insufficient services for the elderly (Gatz et al., 1985).

Intervention experts typically emphasize that treatment should be individualized for the particular client. This is true of older clients as well; age stereotyping may inappropriately shift the focus of treatment from real problems and solutions to what one expects of older persons. The second consideration, then, is that age is only one factor to be considered in individualized treatment. In fact, individual differences within age cohorts are often greater than group differences between older and younger clients (Smyer et al., 1990). It is only a subset of older clients—with highly significant factors, such as memory loss or other major health concerns—for whom age substantially impacts the choice and course of treatment. And for these, it is the attendant features themselves—not age per se—that actually drive the differences.

The authors have observed that some treatment programs are organized around the geriatric status of clientele, often primarily employing support groups. There does seem to be some benefit to older persons when they are grouped with others of similar age, primarily in their level of comfort with the treatment. Such benefits could be easily offset, however, if groups of older persons with diverse problems and needs were treated together or were treated with some standard "older client" approach. In contrast, there are likely different but important benefits to be gained by encouraging intergenerational involvement and reengaging the older client in an expanded and diverse social network.

In spite of their commonalties with younger populations, older adults face particular challenges that could be overlooked if they did not receive sufficient treatment/research emphasis or if clinical assessment did not focus on those challenges. For example, much of the research on bereavement has been done by gerontologists on older populations largely because it is a problem that older persons face more often. Further, this research shows that the context of bereavement may differ in important ways for younger versus older persons. For example, as we discussed in Chapter 2, older bereaved persons are likely to be coping concurrently with a clustering of other stressors, losses, or health events (cf. Hansson, Remondet, & Galusha, 1993). The third point, then, is that older populations may be at greater risk for certain problems. Much of the earlier part of this book examines these vulnerabilities. Therapists who work with older adults must be vigilant for these concerns and sensitive to resulting special needs.

Fourth, age and age-related issues may moderate processes by which difficulties occur and are met. Although treatment processes in older persons are generally similar to those of younger individuals, some processes and treatment outcomes may vary because of age or related circumstances. Age-related differences may affect not only the nature of the problem to be faced, but also the social milieu in which it must be faced. It should come as no surprise that problems and maladaptive patterns are formed and maintained from a variety of conditions, including age-related factors. This variety of contributing factors not only makes understanding psychosocial problems a complex undertaking, but it also yields a rich variety of possible ways in which interventions can be specifically tailored to meet the needs of elderly populations. By attending to the ways in which age-related factors contribute to pathology, we simultaneously highlight opportunities for intervention. Interestingly, we find that one's older status often affects ways in which treatments are applied but is less likely to result in using therapy models that are fundamentally different. For example, older persons are more likely to be treated by older therapists, but the types of psychotherapy employed do not differ from those used with younger patients. Similarly, with older clients, therapy goals are often more limited and hospitalization is more common, but these choices seem to be made for much the same reasons as with younger clients.

TREATMENT OBJECTIVES
VERSUS TREATMENT FOCUS

From the perspective of interpersonal functioning, intervention with older adults can be characterized using a 2 × 2 table, as illustrated in Figure 8.1. First, treatment objectives are divided into two types, relational and nonrelational. Similarly, we split treatment foci into social and nonsocial types. Many interventions focus on directly changing target behaviors or improving target outcomes. However, such direct intervention is often difficult or inefficient. Interventions, therefore, might also be indirect, in that the focus of the actual treatment may be on something associated with or causal to the target outcome. In this case an indirect focus of treatment is usually selected because it is more accessible or easier to change. Because we are specifically interested in the role of relationships and in social functioning, we focus our discussion on interventions in which either the treatment objective is some change in social functioning or the mechanism of intervention is social. Therefore, we now examine three of the four possible intervention approaches shown in Figure 8.1 (quadrants A, B, and C).

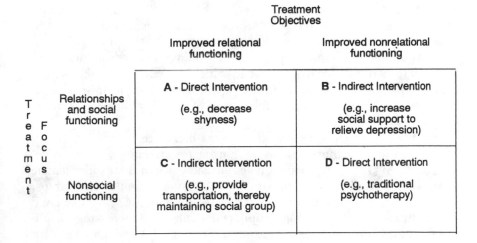

FIGURE 8.1. Intervention and social functioning.

Directly Promoting Positive Social Functioning

Interpersonal functioning is a critical outcome in and of itself: it constitutes a large portion of what is meant by "psychological health" and "general well-being." We seek to directly improve social functioning simply to yield good social functioning (quadrant A). Although this is intuitively obvious, this point is often lost in the effort to relate social functioning to other outcomes. For example, the impetus for much of the work on social support resulted from the finding the support leads to improved health outcomes (e.g., Cohen & Syme, 1985). That social support is satisfying, in itself, is a fact mentioned less often. Similarly, effective social systems, as reflected by positive relationships, effective communication, mutual benefit, and the like can be directly impacted by intervention. We need not look to instrumental outcomes to perceive the improved system as a treatment benefit.

Other Benefits of Good Social Functioning

Although well-being can be arbitrarily divided into "social" functioning and "other" functioning, these two domains are highly related. Nonsocial difficulties can impair interpersonal functioning, just as changes in the social environment can affect nonsocial areas of functioning. Consequently, intervention strategies can be evaluated at the level of the social functioning itself, as described above, or by assessing more general benefits and outcomes linked to relationships and other social functioning, as in quadrant B. The efficacy of this latter treatment is evaluated in terms of nonsocial outcomes, such as health, depression, or mobility, even though the focus of the intervention itself is on directly impacting social functioning. The treatments themselves may not differ from those in which the outcome to be altered is interpersonal; however, the choice of social behavior or attitude to alter is made because of its implications for altering the nonsocial behavior of interest.

Many examples are appearing in the literature of social interventions leading to improvement of nonsocial outcomes. For example, Fredriksen (1992), reporting on an outreach program for older female alcoholics, underscored the importance of building relationships. Among other things, the program focused on building self-esteem and socialization skills, creating a support network, and increasing socialization and participation in organized recreation. Although treatment emphasized social functioning, as intended, control over alcohol was greatly improved for many women.

Nonsocial Interventions That Lead
to Improved Social Functioning

Alternatively, intervention might deal with nonsocial factors that interfere with effective social functioning, as in quadrant C. Examples include modification of living arrangements to increase social contact with the elderly, dealing with one's health or financial limitations to improve mobility and access to social groups, providing support or education to caretakers and family members so they are motivated and able to maintain relationships with the older person, and alleviating depression or other psychiatric conditions that cause withdrawal or interfere with effective interpersonal behavior. Careful analysis of the personal and environmental factors that either interfere with older persons' relationships or maintain dysfunctional behaviors often leads the mental health professional to focus on change in nonsocial areas. In this case, evaluation of success focuses on social functioning, even though treatment does not.

PROBLEMS, OBJECTIVES,
AND TREATMENT PLANNING

Effective interventions require the specification of several factors beyond what is to be done. A host of strategies are available to impact social functioning, and the choice best depends upon achieving a relatively complete understanding of an individual's life situation. We briefly tie together four major areas: problems, objectives and goals of intervention, contextual factors, and the treatment strategies themselves.

Problems

Earlier chapters have alerted the reader to likely areas of interpersonal difficulty for older persons, and there is no need to restate them here. It is worthwhile, however, to note that the specification of a problem requiring intervention is not always easy. Many clients do not present with the most salient, basic, or troubling problem. It is possible that the fundamental concern is outside of awareness or not well enough conceptualized to be communicated. For some it is easier to establish a therapeutic relationship by presenting a difficulty that fits their own definition of being worthy of treatment—for example, one might visit the family physician with vague medical complaints when the real concern is interpersonal (also see Chapter 2).

Relational competence often plays a part in social difficulties and associated conditions among both older and younger persons. However, clients will rarely present with a complaint about their ability to interact with others. For example, the older person may focus on the medical difficulty or financial strain that precipitates a need to interact with social agencies, but he/she may be reluctant to discuss shyness, embarrassment, or communication difficulties that are actually preventing effective interaction with helping agencies. In such cases, focusing on feelings of depression, loneliness, or hopelessness might heighten the older client's sense of vulnerability, whereas working directly on building effective skills for interaction could be empowering. Because the relevance of interpersonal competencies are often not obvious, the importance of a thorough assessment strategy is underscored (see Chapter 6).

Goals

Through much of this book we have discussed areas of social difficulty experienced by older adults generally, as well as the interplay between relationships and overall functioning. Effective intervention, however, is usually individualized and therefore uses this information to identify problems and consider areas most in need of and amenable to change. As problems are identified, it becomes necessary to establish the purposes or goals that are to be achieved. Most problems in the elderly, when viewed from the social/relationship perspective, naturally give rise to several general treatment goals, thereby guiding the intervention. The global purpose of intervention is *to foster social interaction, social support, and positive social attitudes so that the elderly client receives the various social, psychological, and physical benefits of positive interpersonal relations.* Table 8.1 lists several more specific purposes that might be a focus of intervention.

From the perspective of relational competence, goals such as those in Table 8.1 might be viewed as embodying four approaches. First, needed relational skills may be absent, or if present earlier but not recently used, may be atrophied. The goal, then, can be phrased in terms of building or restoring needed social skills and attitudes to effective levels. Second, skills may be present, but the older person does not use them—perhaps because their relevance is not perceived, or because opportunity is limited due to some physical barrier. In this case goals can be phrased in terms of choosing optimum coping strategies, effective utilization of existing skills and resources, and removal of barriers. The third approach emphasizes compensation to substitute for weak or missing competencies. Because relational skills are relatively enduring

TABLE 8.1. Examples of Interpersonal Issues That Might Be a Focus of Intervention

- Maintaining a satisfying level of social interaction in the face of limiting factors related to aging
- Utilizing available support networks to meet new problems arising from old age
- Building or rejuvenating social skills, prosocial attitudes, and socially desirable personality attributes that were less necessary during years of stable work and family relationships but become more necessary as long-standing relationships are lost
- Replacing instrumental relationships lost through factors associated with aging (such as retirement or moving) by increasing other kinds of socializing, engaging in volunteer work, and so forth
- Helping family relationships evolve as the needs of family members change
- Dealing with family and peer group conflict, particularly as novel developmental tasks yield new problems for the relationship
- Creating new expectations and attitudes regarding one's relationships so that the "psychological/perceptual filter" yields positive interpretations and so that motivation regarding reasonable behavior is maintained
- Providing community supports to offset health and social limits resulting from aging
- Providing community supports to family and caretakers to improve quality of care and to prevent caregiver burnout
- Maintaining a level of social involvement that assures one's assets and skills can remain a benefit to the social group

characteristics of the individual, major changes are hard to achieve; however, social competencies serve multiple interpersonal functions, and one might be taught to use existing skills to good advantage even if they are not the most relevant. Finally, the fourth approach recognizes that needed competencies are simply not present at sufficient levels. In this case, rather than building the competence, the intervention provides the functions that would not be met. For example, the shy individual is placed in small social groups so that new contacts are made, the therapist provides a supportive relationship in the absence of supportive others, or a professional arbitrates a family dispute.

Personal and Environmental Factors Precipitating and Maintaining Problems

Typically, a whole constellation of factors come together to support problem behaviors and problem situations. Unfortunately, these factors often go unexplored. Among older adults, these contextual variables are often prominent, are frequently amendable to change, and can play a pivotal role in the development and maintenance of the presenting problem. Indeed, it is not that older adults' problems are unique; rather, the milieu common to many older persons largely justifies studying their relational problems apart from those of younger persons.

Both individual and environmental variables should be considered. For example, an older person might present with a complicated bereavement following the death of the spouse. The depression and loneliness are readily identified as presenting problems and the death as the precipitant. However, increased environmental pressures, such as a shrinking social network due to loss of mobility and limited income, may be less obvious. Similarly, remaining opportunities for interaction may be painful rather than pleasant because of shyness and poor social skill or because the limited nature of these relationships reminds the bereaved person of how much was lost when the spouse died. Intervention might be expanded, then, to include attention to related losses and to enhancement of the intimacy and involvement of previously peripheral relationships.

Family systems therapy and other systems approaches are relevant to this concern. The fundamental concept behind systems approaches is a recognition of the interdependence between one's functioning and one's environment. A change in either impacts the other. Therefore, the systems approach seeks to assess individual functioning as part of the broader system. Thus, contextual features are central to this approach because the therapist seeks to alter the system and not just the individual.

Choice of Intervention and the Treatment Plan

If problems, goals, and context are properly assessed, an intervention strategy naturally follows. Thus, comprehensive evaluation is a prerequisite to treatment planning. Assessment includes, at a minimum, (1) clear delineation of the problem, including duration, frequency, intensity, and manifest behaviors or feelings; (2) evaluation of situational factors that impact it—the context in which the problem occurs; (3) ascertaining important consequences of the problem; (4) understanding functioning within major life domains to ascertain strengths, weaknesses, limits, and opportunities; and (5) reviewing other potential problem areas not encompassed by the focal complaint (to avoid surprises later). As noted by Kane and Kane, " . . . measurements are organizers, capable of turning amorphous and expansive goals into a series of defined tasks. They are the means by which progress or lack of progress is noted" (1981, pp. 1–2). Understanding where a person is and where that person wants to go, along with some notion of his/her capabilities and weaknesses, naturally leads to effective treatment planning.

The treatment plan links together (1) target problems, (2) goals of the treatment, (3) behaviors, attitudes, and environmental factors that are the focus of direct intervention, and (4) mechanisms by which change is to be effected. An effective plan takes the broadly defined goals and intervention strategy to more specific levels, defining intermediate goals, listing the particular relationships to be enhanced and specific social behaviors to be altered, and specifying actions to be taken by the therapist.

RELATIONAL PROBLEMS AND STRESS

Relational Problems as Stressors

Relational problems can be viewed from a number of theoretical perspectives, each leading to interesting intervention approaches. One important perspective, discussed earlier in this volume (Chapters 2 and 7), places relational difficulties within the context of stress and coping. Several parallels exist between social difficulties and stress. For example, the distress of enduring relational difficulties, which is much like a stress reaction, is frequently what leads one to seek professional help. The resources one brings to the relationship determine in large part how one reacts emotionally to pressures, the coping activities chosen to deal with those pressures, and the effectiveness of coping.

In earlier discussions (Carpenter & Scott, 1992; Hansson & Carpenter, 1990) we have emphasized comparisons between stress and relational difficulties (also see Chapter 7). For example, as Hobfoll (1988) noted in his "social ecology" model of stress, proper matching of coping resources and activities to presenting problems most readily leads to stress reduction and effective coping.

Viewing relational difficulties from a stress perspective suggests four obvious points of intervention: (1) resources, (2) perception/reappraisal, (3) stressor, and (4) the stress reaction. Resource intervention takes two main forms, the development of relational competencies and attitudes that contribute to positive relationships and development of a supportive social network. Given the importance of cognitive evaluation both of stressors and of one's ability to cope effectively (Lazarus & Folkman, 1984), interventions that encourage optimistic appraisal of one's circumstances can be effective at reducing negative emotional reactions to relational stressors. Interventions aimed at the social stressors themselves attempt to remove or reduce the source of difficulty; hence, they are often referred to as *problem-focused*. Problem-focused interventions are often emotionally taxing because of the high initial demand on the individual confronting the problem; however, they are often most effective overall because the difficulty is lessened. Finally, interventions aimed at reducing the stress reaction itself, collectively called *emotion-focused,* emphasize relaxation, distraction, and the like. Because some social difficulties cannot be removed, techniques for minimizing their emotional impact can be effective. As we described in Chapter 2, older persons are particularly likely to use emotion-focused coping; skill at such coping may help them perceive less stress in the first place.

Compensatory Control

One of the interesting findings in social-support research is that improved outcomes often result, even if one does not obtain instrumental benefits from the social network. Specifically, a strong support network — or just a belief that others would be supportive if needed — seems to increase resilience, add to a sense of well-being, and encourage active coping. We noted earlier the seemingly paradoxical finding wherein actually receiving support may lead to worse outcomes, apparently because the recipient is reminded of his or her inadequacy or is unable to "take credit" for the favorable outcome (see Box 7.2 for a more complete discussion). These findings serve to underscore the notion that relationships and relational attitudes and characteristics are interwoven into one's self-concept and have significant impact on overall well-being and general coping; outcomes can be affected by relational functioning, even in the absence of direct causal connections.

This application can be applied with considerable potential to the area of personal control. It is well established that a sense of mastery and control over a stressor leads to effective coping, lower physical arousal, and lower sense of threat (e.g., Lefcourt, 1992). We argue that it is appropriate to extend this idea, such that increased control in some areas of functioning can compensate for lowered control in other areas. For example, a person who feels good about his friendships or marriage may have an easier time when pressures at work arise, largely because the former successes lead to a sense of well-being and competence. Thompson (1991) has formalized this idea into a model of compensatory control. She proposes that relationships are a particularly good place to reassert control, an idea with which we agree. In simple terms, if people feel effective in and in control of their relationships, this tends to contribute to overall feelings of mastery and self-esteem that in turn can help the person weather difficulties that have nothing to do with his/her relationships.

MECHANISMS OF INTERVENTION

Intervention strategies are quite diverse, ranging from traditional psychological approaches to manipulations of the client's environment. They have evolved from a number of conceptual models and are relevant to nonsocial as well as social difficulties. We discuss several of the most prevalent here, emphasizing possible applications to relationship difficulties and relational competence.

Individual Psychotherapy

A large number of therapeutic models fall under the general rubric of psychotherapy. Most follow the tradition of individual psychology, focusing on the intrapsychic mechanisms or the behaviors of the individual rather than on the dyad, family, or other social system. The behavioral/learning perspectives tend to consider the social environment primarily as a source of contingencies and reinforcers, whereas more dynamic models treat relationships and significant others mostly as cognitive/emotional constructions of the mind.

In spite of this "individual" orientation, a number of these traditional psychotherapies pay close attention to social functioning, although most treat social interactions as developmental factors affecting identity, cognitive schemas, learned patterns of behaviors, and so forth. For example, Adler's Interpersonal Psychology (1930; Mosak, 1989) examines birth order effects, family patterns of interaction, and communications conveying power structure or acceptance. But in keeping with individual approaches, Adler's model examines this social behavior with an emphasis on predictions about the personality formation and resulting neurotic reactions, such as Adler's "inferiority complex." Consequently, therapists using this model are likely to stress formative social experience or to view current social interaction as reflecting internal states and personality structure ("This is the way *you* are and this is why").

Individual psychotherapies have long been used to help individuals deal with social difficulties (Horowitz & Vitkus, 1986), although the efficacy literature is voluminous and mixed. The authors' impression is that the use of psychotherapy to alleviate relationship problems has shown modest success. Numerous mechanisms probably underlie effectiveness. Psychotherapy might, for example, be particularly effective in shifting attitudes, enhancing motivation, and removing internal/emotional barriers to effective social interaction. However, these results may be too indirect for many relational needs, especially given that psychotherapy is usually time-consuming and costly. In fact, what may often be beneficial about psychotherapy is that the client is afforded a chance to discuss relationships and social problems in detail. This probably yields (1) insight into relational partners or the dynamics of the relationship as much as insight into oneself, (2) information on or models of alternative behavioral patterns, and (3) social support. These nonspecific effects are often not part of the theories underlying many psychotherapies; instead, they perhaps result from the fact that the therapy relationship is itself a special kind of personal relationship (e.g., Derlega, Hendrick, Winstead, & Berg, 1991; Winstead, Derlega, Lewis, & Margulis, 1988).

When the relational problems most common to older clients are considered, such as loss and reduced mobility, the possible limitations of traditional psychotherapies become more evident. For example, many dynamic theories discuss the effects of loss, especially as it influences personality development. However, insight into how the loss of one's spouse of 30 years has contributed to depression, passivity, and dependency may not prove very helpful. Instead, replacement relationships may be most needed.

Finally, writers have noted how difficult it is to significantly change an older person's personality given a relatively longer history (cf., Smyer et al., 1990), while at the same time one advocates brief interventions. This inconsistency has implications for our model of relational competence, in which behavioral repertoires and attitudes are based in relatively enduring individual differences, such as extroversion. Traditional therapies may have a greater potential to alter relatively stable attitudes and behavior patterns, but they probably cannot achieve this under the restraint of brief intervention.

Family Therapy

Family system-based therapies appear to have considerable potential for dealing with relationship difficulties. These approaches are probably good at clarifying needs of group members, improving communication, and solving circumscribed problems facing the group. However, family therapy appears to be underutilized in older populations, especially considering the powerful supportive role often played by the family. Older clients may believe marriage and other family problems to be more pertinent to younger persons, perhaps because they do not recognize that over time their relationships face new developmental tasks (Wolinski, 1986). Also, tradition dictates that family therapy is only for those who live together or for intact families with school-aged children. New attitudes may be necessary to extend this approach to older marriages, adult children and siblings, and family members living apart.

A particular problem may be present when all participants do not live together, in that mutual benefit may not be evident (e.g., the older parent might benefit from more attention from adult children, but the benefit to children is not so readily apparent). Family therapy may be effective at creating motivation by arousing family members' sense of shared responsibility and caring and by exploring solutions that yield relatively equitable roles.

In an interesting study, Thompson and Heller (1990) noted a greater influence on well-being of perceived support from family than from others, at least for older persons who placed high value on family. They concluded that other forms of support may not readily substitute for missing family support for such persons. This is important, given the trend among professionals to deal with disrupted or problematic family relationships by introducing older persons to peers.

Group Therapy

Group therapy is often theoretically similar to individual psychotherapy, but because a group is involved, it emphasizes the benefit of itself being a social system. Groups may be particularly effective at developing social competencies and allowing older adults to try out alternative behavioral patterns (Lieberman, 1983). For example, a positively functioning group provides encouragement and support for exploration of relationship behaviors, with feedback that helps shape effective behaviors. Lieberman and Videka-Sherman (1986) found that positive outcome was related to involvement within the group, however. Thus, those who enter with higher relational competence probably benefit the most. Less skilled participants may require longer participation, initially to foster positive group behaviors and later to achieve more general benefit.

Van Wylen and Dykema-Lamse (1990) described their program for incorporating a group into the daily program of an adult day care center. The similarities in circumstances that brought participants into the day care program suggested common elements on which the group could focus. In particular, Van Wylen and Dykema-Lamse saw the two main difficulties faced by participants as establishing and main-taining meaningful relationships and sustaining self-esteem. Further, participation in the group shifted one's focus from receiving physical care to growth and problem-solving.

It is important to remember that age is only one of many factors and may not be the best criterion for group formation. Group cohesiveness and homogeneity are critical to successful group functioning, and these are more likely to arise in groups with a shared therapeutic agenda. Also, a number of studies underscore the importance of assuring that the relational skill level of participants is sufficiently high to lead to positive and productive exchanges (e.g., Timko & Moos, 1990). Thus, a homogeneous but low-functioning group, even with a capable group leader, may not be able to facilitate productive exchange.

Social Skills Training and Other Behavioral Models

For many older persons, a primary barrier to adaptation to age-related change in their social environment is a lack of adequate social skills. Training new skills is therefore a natural and effective reaction to inadequate relational competencies. We generally view relational competence as involving relatively enduring dispositions and attitudes of the individual. It would not be inconsistent, however, for learned skills to enhance the effectiveness of one's global characteristics (an extraverted person may be comfortable meeting new people but may be overbearing or clumsy) or to help compensate for limitations.

Although not required by the underlying model, social skills training historically has tended to emphasize assertive behavior and skills for meeting new people, especially as they apply to young adults. A number of approaches have successfully adapted these approaches to older populations (e.g., Engels, 1991; Smyer et al., 1990). For example, Franzke (1987) provided assertiveness training to a group of elders. Her 6-week course yielded improvements in both assertive behavior and self-concept. Social skills training with older adults is usually traditional in form (e.g., role playing and behavioral assignments), but the content can be expanded to social behaviors not found in many social-skills groups, such as intimacy-enhancing behaviors.

In the past, skills programs focused primarily on young adult populations. Thus, adaptations to contexts and situations relevant to elderly persons have been an important trend. For example, Shulman and Mandel (1988) report on a program to improve communication between institutionalized elders and their family and friends. The relatives and friends learned about how aging impacts communication and learned skills for keeping communication open and productive, resulting in improved relationships and increased satisfaction with visits.

It appears that other behavioral models can be readily adapted to meet the social needs of elderly clients. For example, social learning theory suggests that older adults can learn from others who face similar relationship difficulties, especially when these others model effective behavior.

Community Interventions

One of the most effective interventions is to provide opportunities for meaningful relationships. A forum for interacting with others, especially when built around a shared interest, facilitates the development of satisfying friendships. Organizing groups around a particular focus provides an agenda for discourse and acquaintance building. With limitations on mobility and income, or because of other factors that encourage isolation, some elderly persons may not readily develop their own social groups (see Chapter 3). Thus, community support for a variety of groups can facilitate this process. This support might include financial support, providing a meeting place, offering resources such as equipment, interesting speakers or experts on the topic of group focus, and providing information, expertise, or leadership for organizing groups. Once such groups are initiated, they are often self-perpetuating.

Cox and Parsons (1992) describe an interesting community intervention in which relationally skilled older persons were given special training to allow them to help others. In their program older volunteers were taught mediation skills. These lay mediators then assisted other seniors in resolving of conflicts, such as with housing, consumer problems, or family problems.

Another form of community intervention is the support group. These are similar to therapy groups, but they focus less on change and professional leadership (Lieberman, 1987). Older persons with shared difficulties learn from each other, find strength from group membership, and are able to normalize their concerns, often without the need for professional involvement.

A fair amount of attention has recently focused on support offered by those *not* in an ongoing relationship with the elderly person, with mixed results (e.g., Heller, Thompson, Trueba, & Hogg, 1991). In this approach the recipient, usually an older person at some elevated risk due to health or immobility, receives substitute social support through telephone contacts or brief home visits. The mixed findings for these interventions may result because they provide more instrumental benefit than social benefit.

Instrumental Interventions

We have seen that reduced social functioning in older persons can result from nonsocial factors that limit involvement. It is not surprising, therefore, that instrumental interventions are often effective. These interventions take a wide variety of forms, including transportation, improved health care, community commitment to keep up neighborhoods in which elderly persons live, and financial support.

Morrow-Howell and Ozawa (1987) describe one such program in which elderly volunteers were trained to provide both instrumental and emotional support to their neighbors. The volunteers made telephone contact to provide reassurance, socialized with those that were home-bound, and helped with shopping and transportation. Because of their regular contact, they were also in a good position to assess special needs and refer to professionals before problems became severe.

Recent research has also begun to explore how housing and the tasks of daily living improve or inhibit positive social interaction. Although many factors contribute to an optimum living arrangement for older persons, social factors are gaining in importance. Timko and Moos (1990) found, for example, that greater interpersonal support and self-direction occur when facilities are well equipped, are not too large and impersonal, have policies that encourage autonomy, and residents are socially competent. This issue is explored in greater detail in Chapter 9.

As we saw in Chapters 3 and 4, another concern is the discontinuity in relationships that occurs when older persons must move into residential care. A clear trend is the development of programs, often much less costly than residential care, that provide home care and postpone moves to nursing home (e.g., Berman, Delaney, Gallagher, Atkins, & Graeber, 1987).

We have noted that fear of crime among older persons is often significant and is associated with problems in social functioning, such as shyness and negative perceptions both of the neighborhood and of the availability of helping resources (Hansson & Carpenter, 1986). Similarly, Krause (1991) found that life stressors, including fear of crime and financial strain were associated with distrust and self-imposed isolation. Community efforts to make older neighborhoods safer might help prevent withdrawal and allow older persons to remain in their homes longer, although we suspect that personal tendencies toward withdrawal may also contribute to a perception of an unsafe environment.

Finally, caregivers—usually family members—frequently have considerable demands placed on them by the deteriorating health or cognitive impairment of older care recipients (see Chapter 4). Community supports for caregivers may increase their resilience and prolong their ability to successfully care for the elderly person. These supports can take the form of caregiver training, compensation programs to offset lost income and other expenses of caregiving, substitute caregivers to allow time off, and home-based professional help to meet special needs that the caregiver cannot provide. For example, Knight, Lutzky, and Macofsky-Urban (1993) reviewed studies of the effectiveness of respite care and found consistent benefit for caregivers, usually greater than that achieved through caregiver support groups. Berman et al. (1987) provide a good example of a respite program. Their program supplied brief inpatient care as needed to relieve caregivers and also provided training in care delivery and help in building other community supports. They found such respite care not only supported the in-home caregiver, but it also prevented premature removal of the elderly patient to long-term care facilities. Recognizing that the caregiver is often the most important relational partner underscores the need to keep that relationship vital (Zarit, 1990).

SUMMARY

A variety of intervention strategies appear to be feasible for working with older adults. However, interventions should emphasize individualized treatment, paying attention to those problems that are common among elderly clients but at the same time understanding that age is only one of many factors likely to shape needed treatment.

The roles of relational functioning and interpersonal competence are not always evident from presenting problems. A systematic evaluation of the interpersonal domain is therefore essential. Opportunities for interventions in social functioning are varied, often also impacting and being affected by nonsocial functioning. Direct interventions include building skills, developing strategies for effective use of skills, learning to compensate for behavioral weaknesses, work with family, peers, or other social networks, and supportive therapy. Indirect interventions might include optimizing social access, alleviating medical and psychological conditions that interfere, and improving availability of helping agencies.

Understanding the older person's relational competencies involves an assessment of strengths and weaknesses critical to the relational tasks currently challenging the older client. This leads to treatment strategies in which needed interpersonal skills are built, areas of relational difficulty are anticipated, strengths are used to solve social problems, and areas are highlighted for which external support and compensation will be required.

CHAPTER 9

SPECIAL PROBLEMS OF THE ELDERLY: DEPRESSION, HOUSING, LEGAL INCOMPETENCE, AND CAREGIVER STRAIN

I n this chapter we examine four particular problems that impact and are impacted by social functioning and relational competence. There is nothing unique about the problems selected. They are common concerns and have been briefly discussed in earlier portions of this book. However, with the information provided by earlier chapters (about relationship problems, functioning in the elderly, relational competence, and intervention), the reader is prepared to analyze relational concerns of the elderly. The problems discussed here were chosen because they often strongly impact the elderly person and because they are prototypes of other difficulties commonly encountered in elderly groups needing psychological or medical intervention. The reader, then, is encouraged to think beyond the problem discussed to other difficulties of a similar type, generalizing the ideas and methods proposed. For example, our discussion of depression in large measure applies to other psychiatric difficulties, such as anxiety and dementia.

In keeping with the theme of this book, we attempt to turn the reader's attention to social factors and to the individual's relational competencies. However, we also try to introduce other factors—such as health and health delivery, biology, finances, and legal issues—that place these issues within a proper context. Effective assessment and intervention typically require attention to all facets of elders' problems, not just to the interpersonal. Hopefully, our discussion sets a proper example.

DEPRESSION

Depression is a particularly serious problem for the elderly. Like many of the age-related difficulties we have examined, depression has a variety of causes and consequences. When it occurs, regardless of the reason, it tends to interfere with relationships. Similarly, those with relational deficits seem especially vulnerable. Because of its significance, we examine this problem in extra detail and discuss ways in which relational competence and social interventions can help older adults deal with it.

Prevalence, Course, and Causes

Depression appears to be the most prevalent psychological disorder among the elderly, and older persons represent a particularly vulnerable age group for this disorder. Prevalence estimates of depressed mood among the elderly run at about 15%–20%, and perhaps as high as 25% among institutionalized elderly (Blazer, Hughes, & George, 1987; Fry, 1986; Parmelee, Katz, & Lawton, 1992). It is not clear if the prevalence of diagnosable major depression is substantially higher for older than for younger persons, and some have concluded that depression in the elderly is more a function of associated conditions of aging rather than aging per se (e.g., Cappeliez, 1988). As with younger populations, older women are at considerably higher risk for being diagnosed with clinical depression than are older men (although this appears, in part, to be because of differences in willingness to seek treatment).

For most victims, depression is episodic, with relatively normal functioning between episodes. However, 20%–35% of depressives may have more chronic forms, without marked episodes or with substantial residual impairment between episodes. Among those receiving a diagnosis of major depression, most will have two or more episodes, although few will have more than about four to six. The average age for the first bout with clinical depression is around 40, reflecting the fact that many people are first affected in their older years. In patients with multiple depressive episodes, the recovery period tends to become shorter with age, even though the episodes themselves tend to be as long as before. Thus, as such individuals age, they are depressed more of the time. This is also true for individuals who first develop depression relatively late in life; they too often have shorter symptom-free intervals than do younger patients. Finally, episodes later in life are often more severe and have more acute onset, a pattern suggestive of biological causes; similarly, major life events seem to play a smaller role in triggering an episode (Gold, Goodwin, & Chrousos, 1988).

As with younger persons, the causes for depression among the elderly are varied and complex. It seems that the increase in depression with age probably reflects two classes of age-related developments, biological changes and functional decline. In older adults, biological causes for depression often appear prominent. For example, sleep and other biological rhythm disturbances are common to older persons and to depressed persons. In addition, there is substantial symptom similarity between depression and some other disorders common to older persons, especially dementia, making differential diagnosis a problem. These often chronic, limiting health conditions no doubt lead to symptoms characteristic of depression, such as withdrawal, feelings of helplessness and hopelessness, and reduction in pleasant activities; thus, persons with such chronic conditions are often also depressed (e.g., Williamson & Schulz, 1992). The intertwined nature of such health problems and depression is characterized by Fry (1986):

> Since many elderly have somatic and organic complaints and often also show sadness, their symptoms should not automatically be dismissed merely as signs of depression or merely as part of the normal aging process. Most elderly have at least one chronic illness or health problem and have numerous somatic complaints that might present symptoms of depression. Hence the task of differentiating normal from pathological symptomatology becomes a difficult but important one for the clinician or practitioner. (p. 78)

Notice that Fry also suggests a tendency for some clinicians to "normalize" depression in older persons to the point of disregarding it. In fact, most older adults are in good mental health (e.g., Busse, 1987), reminding us that depression may be common but is not inevitable. Given the impact of depression on elders' quality of life, and given a high rate of treatment success, a casual attitude toward depression is unwarranted.

Some writers emphasize the increasing role of biology among the causes for elderly depression, which the evidence seems to support (Gold et al., 1988). However, environmental factors are probably still prominent (e.g., Blazer, Burchett, Service, & George, 1991). For example, a major cause of depressed mood in the elderly is bereavement (normal bereavement is not diagnosed as major depression in DSM-III-R). Further, the impact of environment may often be more subtle because many negative factors contributing to depression tend to shift with age from discrete life events to chronic stressors. Indeed, models of stress in the elderly (see Chapters 6 and 7) emphasize depression as an important outcome of the stress process.

In a longitudinal study of adults age 65 or older, Russell and Cutrona (1991) tested a model of how social support, life events, and daily hassles (smaller but usually chronic demands) contribute to later depression. They found that social support predicted current and future depression and predicted daily hassles. However, unlike common findings with younger subjects, life events were not predictive of later depression, although daily hassles were. Similarly, Keith (1987) studied older and younger couples and found that job and life strains were more closely linked to depressive symptomatology among younger couples. At the same time, his data underscored the presence of relational difficulties among those who were depressed, but not among the nondepressed. These and other studies suggest, then, that major life stresses are not the main environmental contributors to depression in the elderly. However, this does not mean that stress models or other models that propose an important causal role for environment are not valid for older adults. Rather, we continue to see an important role for social support and relationships, as well as for stressors of a more chronic nature.

Intervention and Prevention

Because of the reciprocal nature of social functioning and depression, it is useful to examine intervention and prevention from two perspectives, depression as a contributor to relational dysfunction and poor social functioning as a contributor to depression. With this in mind, we make four general recommendations.

First, assessment of the elderly should pay particular attention to the possibility of depression. It is important to discard stereotypes such as (1) depressive symptoms are a normal consequence of aging, and (2) such symptoms cannot or need not be treated. Direct intervention on depression is useful for maintaining positive relational functioning that is critical for well-being, independence, and other positive outcomes. Hence, it is critical to accurately diagnose depression and underlying conditions that contribute to depressive symptomatology.

There are some older persons at special risk who will often not present to a physician or therapist for diagnosis, perhaps because of isolation, confusion, or a lack of appreciation that their condition is treatable. Several communities have developed programs to pay special attention to older adults living independently and alone. Such programs may include regular assessment visits by mental health workers. Alternatively, non-mental health workers in frequent contact with the public (such as utility workers) can be taught warning signs of elder distress (such as lack of communication or loss of personal hygiene) and how to make referrals for follow-up by professionals (e.g., Gurian,

1992). These programs, in effect, establish a support network for individuals who would otherwise not have one.

Our second recommendation is that traditional treatment for depression should be vigorously pursued with older clients. The value of remediation is especially marked for older adults—not only is reduction in depression a valuable benefit, but improvement should also help reduce risks for outcomes associated with depression for which older persons are already at elevated risk (e.g., suicide, decline in quality of life, and damage to fragile existing relationships important for preserving remaining autonomy). Research clearly shows that traditional treatments for depression are effective for elderly patients (e.g., Gaylord & Zung, 1987; Thompson et al., 1987). However, traditional approaches applied to the older adult are not without special challenges. For example, use of antidepressive medication often results in unexpected side effects, perhaps because of age-related changes in brain functioning, blood flow, renal functioning, and the like (Fry, 1986; Gaylord & Zung, 1987). With psychotherapy, there are the special challenges mentioned in Chapter 8, such as therapist biases, the reluctance of older clients to seek treatment, and better outcomes for time-limited and focused approaches.

Although not obvious from the treatment literature for depression among elders, we propose that relationship enhancement can be an important intervention. As we have discussed earlier, weak support or loss of support is important in the development of depression. Similarly, supportive, group, and family therapies often help. However, most therapies do not tap the full spectrum of possibilities regarding enhancement of relational functioning. An integrated approach could include: offering professional or peer support, enhancing friendships and family relationships, introducing the depressed client to new social groups, providing activities with a social component, and training needed social skills.

In addition to intervention after the onset of depression, targeting vulnerable individuals for preventive support is often a valuable and efficient approach. Our third recommendation, then, is that we use our knowledge of risk variables (especially relational risk variables) to target elderly persons vulnerable to depression. Often community programs that target elderly persons for special attention define "at risk" in ways that include those likely to develop depression. For example, common risk variables include living alone, having poor health, and having previously interacted with social service agencies. Based on relationship research, we can also recommend attention to persons who: recently experienced loss of a family member, have poor relationship skills, recently made a change in living arrangement, and have diminished mobility. As emphasized throughout this book, those with poor relational competence are most likely to have and be affected by social difficulties; thus, we think that determining who is at risk requires assessment of one's relational competence for the particular social challenges at hand.

After targeting at risk individuals, our fourth recommendation is that we compensate for and reduce weaknesses that make these persons vulnerable. Professionals interacting with the elderly should not wait for the development of depression but should promote positive relational functioning as a buffer against depression. Although this can take much the same form as intervention described above, it will usually not be in the form of individual, group, or family therapy. One form with proven effectiveness is increasing social support, such as through peer support (e.g., Cox & Parsons, 1992; Kirkpatrick & Patchner, 1987; Ong, Martineau, Lloyd, & Robbins, 1987; Scharlach, 1988), contact with community agencies, and maintaining the viability of family supports (e.g., see below for a discussion of supporting family caregivers).

RELATIONSHIPS AND HOUSING

Age-related limitations and needs have prompted many to propose ways for optimizing the environment for the elderly (e.g., Parmelee & Lawton, 1990). For example, Rowles (1987) proposes that housing can be aligned along a continuum of independence to dependence. Such an alignment is very similar to the model we proposed in Chapter 5 for social functioning (Tables 5.1 and 5.3), underscoring the intertwined nature of housing needs and relationships. At the independent end of Rowles' continuum, where one lives in standard community housing, such as single-family homes, the resident has high independence but must be able to function with that independence. As the need for support increases, autonomy is sacrificed through housing options that make help more convenient but remove choices. Parmelee and Lawton (1990) propose that these issues are characterized by two, often competing, goals—autonomy and security. As security needs increase (such as the need for health security resulting from growing frailty), meeting those needs may require moving to a setting in which some elements of choice and autonomy are relinquished.

The interpersonal elements of living arrangements are substantial, and often contribute to the environment's functional adequacy and satisfaction level. For example, Dean, Kology, Wood, and Matt (1992) found that older persons who live alone experience greater depressive symptomatology, even after controlling for support from friends, life events, disability, and financial strain. Further, those living alone seemed more negatively affected by the onset of substantial health problems than did those living with others. In a study of 725 elderly persons, la Gory and Fitzpatrick (1992) also found that environmental factors, including the availability of social support and the degree to which neighbors are also elderly, were associated with depression.

Living with Other Elders

The advantages and disadvantages of age-homogeneous housing suggest some interesting applications of relationship concepts. For example, living with other elders typically yields greater satisfaction with housing (e.g., George, 1987). Thus, those in retirement communities enjoy having maximal opportunity to relate to others of their own age. Activities in such communities are geared to the common interests of older persons. Also, the variety of possible relational partners is increased, perhaps minimizing the negative impact of any weaknesses in relationship-initiating competencies. Greater time freedom among many retired persons likely allows friends and neighbors to be an effective support network (interestingly, some studies point to positive benefits of *giving* support, e.g., Krause, 1987). Further, other elders may be more knowledgeable and empathic about age-related difficulties, motivating them to be more supportive and allowing emotional support to be more effective.

There do appear to be some potential drawbacks to age-homogeneous housing, however. Most notably, a setting might become overloaded with frail, needy elderly, with an insufficient base of high-functioning older persons to offer support and maintain a positive environment. This is what seems to happen in some older neighborhoods, where financial and functional limitations among residents eventually interfere with efforts to prevent deterioration of housing; consequently, high-functioning persons stay away, and crime or other undesirable elements may encroach. Similarly, in medical care facilities such a large proportion of residents may be low-functioning ones that close relationships don't develop, and only professional staff are able to provide much support.

Finally, many positive settings designed especially for elders are expensive, putting them out of the reach of most senior citizens. Parmelee and Lawton (1990) point out that over the last decade government support has waned for housing designed for the elderly. Thus, financial and other barriers (e.g., reluctance to leave the family home) mean that many seniors will find themselves living apart from other elders and will need alternative opportunities to interact with peers.

Staying at Home

Several writers have noted the importance of "home"—as opposed to just "housing"—for older adults who find other elements of their security and past slipping away (e.g., Rowles, 1987). This desire for sameness and a sense of security means that many persons will resist relocation as they age, perhaps even if much of what that home used to mean to them, such as family and neighbors, has already been lost. A decade ago Lawton and Hoover (1981) found that about 85% of all older people live in ordinary homes in ordinary communities, and about 75% of these own their homes. For these people, the pull to stay in the same home gives them little control over who their neighbors are. We anticipate, then, that those who are able to develop relationships within the broader social environment will find the greatest satisfaction with their living arrangements and will resist declines associated with weak support systems.

If supportive neighbors are lacking, three other forms of relationships appear important. First, family can offset much of the loss that often occurs as the older person's neighborhood changes, especially if family members live with the older person. When younger family remains close by and provides assistance, tasks that become challenging (such as lawn care, major home repairs, and shopping) are still manageable. Second, relationships in the broader community, including friendships and participation in clubs or religious groups, can provide instrumental support and meaningful social ties. Participation in some of these may require mobility, although some communities have special transportation programs that help. Third, given the benefit to the older person, as well as cost savings to communities, it is in the community's best interest to provide professional and community supports to allow those older persons in vulnerable settings to remain independent as long as possible. Home visits by geriatric nurses or mental health workers, home nursing care for temporary conditions or partial home nursing care for chronic conditions, instrumental supports like Meals on Wheels, neighbor-to-neighbor programs, and brief hospitalization programs all are designed to compensate for limited or transient weaknesses that might otherwise force older persons from their homes and into nursing homes.

Moving to New Housing

In spite of efforts to remain independent and at home, many will be unable to do so because of functional limitations or the need for ongoing health care. When moves occur it is always challenging to develop new relationships, and is often more so for older persons who have spent most of their later life in long-term relationships. Those who plan for a change, rather than waiting until declines force it upon them, will often make the transition better because their functional level is usually still high. With better functioning, it will tend to be easier for them to establish themselves socially in the new setting. Also, if such moves are made with spouses or they are able to maintain old relationships after moves, they bring an important social buffer with them that helps support them until new relationships develop. Once again, relational competence will play an important role in one's success.

Some communities for older persons have built into their design easy transition from independent to supportive environments, with minimal loss of relationships. Within the same setting are included independent apartments or homes, along with partial care and nursing care facilities; also included are activity programs and most basic services, such as lawn care, food services, and medical support. The functional young-old have a relatively easy time developing new relationships in this age-homogeneous environment, and if they later experience declines, most supports are available without requiring a move. If a move to a partial- or full-nursing care facility is required, their friendships, their familiar surroundings, and most of their routine can remain intact. Unfortunately, such well-designed settings must necessarily be done on a large scale and are relatively expensive, making them somewhat scarce and available to only a limited group of seniors. In addition (as we described in Chapter 3), increasing frailty often results in unintended disruptions of one's relationships with younger, healthier residents and in stressful encounters with staff.

For those relocating to nursing homes and hospitals, persons with greater relational skills may more rapidly develop new relationships, although they may also experience greater loss from the move because of the relatively greater importance to them of their relational ties (cf. Tesch, Nehrke, & Whitbourne, 1989). A number of programs have, however, shown that institutions can ease the transition by attending to social needs. For example, volunteers trained to function as network builders can promote morale and meet relational needs (Korte & Gupta, 1991), and communication skills training for residents' friends and families can improve the quality of visits (Shulman & Mandel, 1988). Similarly, nursing home staff can meet relationship needs to some extent. In one program, noncaregiving staff each befriended one resident, providing residents with an additional tie to the outside, an advocate within the setting, and increased self-esteem (Moss & Pfohl, 1988).

COMPETENCE AND GUARDIANSHIP

In Chapter 4 we introduced a variety of concerns regarding guardianship arrangements for elderly persons. About 80% of all guardianships involve older adults, and the number of guardianships is increasing rapidly. Clearly, there are some for whom guardianship is a sensible option. However, researchers find that procedures and outcomes may often be motivated by factors other than the best interest of the elderly ward (e.g., Bulcroft et al., 1991). Most guardians are family members, and the courts appear to assume that this assures an effort to "protect" and serve the older ward. Courts appear to routinely grant petitions with little subsequent oversight or provisions for review, even though research suggests that incompetence is frequently not demonstrated, family actions are often motivated by interest in preserving the estate, and role conflict of guardians is often present (Alexander & Lewin, 1972; Bulcroft et al., 1991; Iris, 1988). Full rather than partial guardianship is nearly always the result, and almost no wards ever have rights restored, even though declines that might lead to incapacity are often limited in scope and variable in course. Thus, in addition to competence, guardianship involves a variety of general relationship issues, such as family conflict, decision-making processes, and the relational stress that sometimes accompanies aging within other contexts.

Because guardianship is determined through legal proceedings, where change is needed it must come mostly through legal channels. However, guardianship is usually initiated by family, so family norms make it hard to protest. Having one's family institute proceedings may engender self-doubt in still competent older persons. Legitimate limitations that do not deprive the elder of judgment or of the ability to handle most concerns can still leave the person vulnerable to family pressure. Even when the elderly person does protest, it is usually informal, and almost none seek independent legal representation. Nonlegal professionals working with older adults, such as mental health workers and medical personnel, would seem ideally suited to assume an advocacy role on this matter. In some states such professionals are already involved in advising the court and can therefore impact specific cases. We believe it is useful for readers of this book to be aware of this issue.

We suspect that relational competence and positive relationships can play a significant role in this process. First, social competencies are part of the overall competencies that should drive decisions about the ability of older adults to independently manage their affairs. As standards and procedures evolve in this area, as they have in other domains of legal competency (e.g., competence to stand trial, including the ability to work with one's attorney; Nicholson & Kugler, 1992), older persons with greater relational competence will likely be more functional and less often adjudicated incompetent. Emerging assessment procedures, like those we propose in Chapters 6 and 8, may contribute to better ways of evaluating competence.

Second, except in the most severe forms of cognitive incapacitation or health failure, help with one's limitations is probably sufficient, leaving the older person to make most of his/her own decisions (e.g., Wilber, 1991). Assistance to overcome limitations may involve community supports, but it can often be provided by family and friends. Obviously, those older persons with the most supportive relationships are best equipped to meet limitations and handle their affairs without creating excessive concern in others.

Finally, it is a concern that factors other than the status of the older adult sometimes motivate guardianship petitions. This suggests that dysfunctional family functioning also may be an issue. In this case the relational functioning of the entire family is relevant. Positive relational skills could help families to resolve family conflict, promote family cohesion (so that feelings about inheritance do not overcome these values), and handle caregiving responsibilities in ways that minimize resentment. We suspect that those who attend to positive family relationships throughout their lives will promote attitudes in their family that deter selfish motives.

CAREGIVERS AND CAREGIVER STRAIN

Even though many problems involving elderly persons arise from family conflict, abuse, and selfishness, many family members provide great service to their older relatives. As increasing frailty requires increasing levels of support and care, it is usually family members who provide it. In Chapter 4 we outlined difficulties that arise because of the stresses of caregiving, both for the caregiver and the recipient. Whether or not a caregiver is a family member, this special relationship is particularly valuable for maintaining independence and well-being of those with substantial limitations (e.g., Bass & Noelker, 1987; Zarit, Birkel, & Malone Beach, 1989). Studies routinely point to the importance of community care for keeping frail adults out of more expensive and confining settings, such as hospitals and nursing homes. For example, Pearlman and Crown (1992) found that having a family caregiver or a caregiver of long duration (emphasizing the relational components) was effective for keeping at-risk persons in home care and out of nursing homes.

Although relational functioning of both the caregiver and recipient are important, in many chronic-care situations in which cognitive capacities or speech are greatly reduced (as in cases of advanced Alzheimer disease or severe stroke), the caregiver will be the main contributor. We here highlight three main ways in which relational competence is relevant to caregiver situations. First, effective relational functioning can help make the caregiver–recipient relationship a positive and meaningful one. This is particularly important to many older adults receiving care, in that the limitations and frailty contributing to their need for care often also cause their other relationships to diminish. It is important to remember, however, that with the pressures of caregiving demands, often with a need for the caregiver to be continually available and vigilant, caregivers themselves can become isolated (Skaff & Pearlin, 1992). We suspect that elderly care recipients who are relationally skilled, especially with enhancement skills, are better able to promote closeness, communicate their needs and their appreciation for care, and play an emotionally contributing role in giver–recipient relationships. Positive contributions to the relationship help offset the imbalance in instrumental contributions. Similarly, relationally skilled caregivers will work better with care recipients, attend better to the older person's relational needs, promote an association that will be positive for both giver and recipient, and deal more effectively with relationship issues that usually arise in chronic care situations (e.g., disagreement, resistance, and embarrassment).

Second, relational competence contributes to better care. Care recipients who are thoughtful, open, and warm probably receive somewhat better care, on the average, because their relationship skills promote a positive association in which the caregiver is motivated to be caring and conscientious. Even though caregiving is stressful and often limits the caregiver's options, helping someone you truly like probably reduces resentment, resistance, and the probability of caregiver burnout. Similarly, skilled caregivers will be better at calming, supporting, negotiating with, and communicating with the elderly care recipient. Such skills may be especially relevant when the patient is socially unskilled, combative, frightened, resistant, or confused. In fact, the presence of enhancement attributes — such as love, sense of duty, and caring — are important reasons why caregivers initially agree to provide care (Guberman, Maheu, & Maille, 1992).

Third, relational functioning is important for helping the caregiver. The recent literature emphasizes the demands placed on the caretaker, and the stress of caregiving is well documented (Dura, Stukenberg, & Kiecolt-Glaser, 1991; Gatz, Bengtson, & Blum, 1990). The potential isolation of caregivers becomes particularly important when we consider caregiving from a stress perspective (cf., Barusch, 1988; Hinrich-

sen, 1991; Pruchno & Kleban, 1993). As in other stress research, social support is a powerful variable for offsetting caregiver stress (e.g.,
Vitaliano, Russo, Young, Teri, & Maiuro, 1991). Thus, caregivers
most able to maintain and use outside relationships appear to handle
caregiver demands the best. They involve other family, effectively use
community support, and derive resilience from their relationships.

In keeping with this, interventions for stressed caregivers focus
on providing support. In a review of 10 years of studies, Knight et
al. (1993) found that supportive interventions were effective. Instrumental support, such as community respite programs that give the family
caretaker time off, are especially helpful. For example, Berman et al.
(1987) found that as-needed hospital respite care replenished caregiver
resilience and reduced early institutionalization, and Mohide et al.
(1990) found that weekly in-home respite care reduced caregiver
depression.

Similarly, interventions that provide emotional support reduce
caregiver distress (Knight et al., 1993). For example, Goodman and
Pynoos (1988) described a telephone network of caregivers, whereas
Toseland, Rossiter, Peak, and Smith, (1990) and Robinson (1988)
found more traditional group and individual skills/coping therapies
helpful for reducing caregiver distress. Caregiver support and education groups have been found to even reduce institutionalization rates
(Greene & Monahan, 1987).

Finally, some programs provide information support. For example, Sheehan (1989) described a program in which religious and social service providers were trained in caregiver issues and ways of
providing information to caregivers. The program improved knowledge
about aging and caregiving and stimulated the development of caregiver
programs. Halpert (1988) found similar success having volunteer organizations provide caregiver information to rural family caregivers.
Penning and Wasyliw (1992) describe a program that makes individualized learning modules, an audiovisual library, and peer counseling
available to caregivers and care recipients in their homes, thereby en-
riching their lives.

CHAPTER 10

CONCLUDING THOUGHTS

We noted at the outset that later life is a time of critical transitions. Aging successfully requires continual adaptation to change within the individual, the family, and the broader environment. We noted also the many ways in which personal relationships and the various components of an older adult's social-care system can enhance adaptation and well-being generally. For most people, these processes and social relationships serve long and well. At times, however, they can be problematic. In this context, a number of broader themes deserve emphasis.

First, we believe that the older adult should be viewed as (and encouraged to be) an active player in the process, able to initiate and enhance supportive personal relationships until very late in life. What the individual brings to the situation in terms of social skills and dispositions can change the odds of successfully constructing, accessing, and maintaining these relationships.

Second, our reading of the research and clinical literatures and our own work suggest that people (of any age) exhibit enduring individual differences in relational competence. In a stable and supportive environment, even those older individuals who are low in relational competence may continue to adapt well to age-related change. Upon the loss or deterioration of that supportive environment, however, their range of adaptive potential may be quite limited.

Third, aging must be viewed in its complexity. It involves physical, psychological, and social change at the level of the individual. It encompasses a clustering of losses and demands for new forms of coping and adaptation. However, it also affects the structure and functioning of the family. It is embedded within the traditions of our social, economic, and political institutions as society imposes age-related rights, obligations, eligibility markers, and a "social clock" by which we are often judged. Aging shades the perceptions of family members, health practitioners, legal systems (and even older persons themselves) regarding an older adult's status, competence, and potential for self-direction and independence. It may deny us the opportunity for full, reciprocal participation in our relationships, resulting in relational strain or loss. Any professional working with older persons and the issues that concern them must also appreciate and accommodate this complexity. We note with encouragement, therefore, that gerontological researchers and clinicians have devoted considerable attention to the development of strategies and instruments for multidimensional assessments of older adults, their problems, and their available coping resources.

Fourth, older persons are first and foremost individuals. Older populations are increasingly heterogeneous within many of the most important domains of their lives. Nevertheless, there do appear to be important age-related changes in the tasks faced by individuals and in the kinds of physical, economic, and social coping resources they may have available. We have attempted (in Chapter 5 of this volume) to impose a conceptual structure on these changes in such a way as to suggest the interplay among (1) age-related events/coping demands, (2) the likely nature of available social support/caregiving, (3) the likely status of potentially supportive social networks, (4) relational challenges likely to arise given one's status on the previous variables, and (5) those aspects of relational competence likely to become important at such a time. The structure of this model provides a basis for integrating and understanding currently available research and for thinking about future research priorities.

As we noted in Chapter 7, however, research on relational competence to date has unevenly addressed the age-related, relational challenges delineated in our model (Table 5.3). Much of the research we have discussed has focused either on the relational challenges characteristic of the early portions of the model, where the individual retains considerable competence with which to cope, or on relational challenges that impact all age groups, such as the need to make new friends. In contrast, very little attention has been paid to the role of relational competence very late in life, when the relational challenges involve more serious health declines and adjustments to greater levels of dependency on support networks, institutions whose primary focus is medical, guardianship arrangements, and so on. One of our major goals in this book was to try to capture the broad scope of age-related concerns in the relationships of older adults, to examine patterns of increasing dependency, and to anticipate the implications for relational competence at each broad stage of dependency. During our early reviews of potentially relevant literatures, we discovered again and again relational competence issues in contexts that had never occurred to us (e.g., see the discussion of guardianship issues and abuses in Chapter 4). We were pleasantly reminded by such events of how the integrative process inevitably produces anomalies and surprises that force the investigator to take the next conceptual step.

Fifth, the model presented in Chapter 5 also provides leads for those charged with planning interventions with the elderly, their families, and social care systems. Responsible interventions (as we noted in Chapters 7 and 8) can only follow an assessment-based identification of (1) the problem and the context in which it occurs, (2) the consequences of the problem, and (3) the individual's strengths, weaknesses, limits, and opportunities.

Finally, there remains much to be done. There are glaring holes in the literature regarding the family/caregiver systems of the elderly, the dynamics of family systems as the time approaches to intervene in the affairs of an older parent, and the potential of older adults to negotiate and assert their needs and rights within our social institutions. More research is also needed to broadly explore individual differences (e.g., in coping style or in relational competence) that older adults bring to the situation, and to assess the efficacy of training, support, or therapeutic interventions with older persons and their families. Fortunately, researchers and practitioners from many disciplines (gerontology, medicine, and the social and behavioral sciences more generally) continue to examine these issues from many perspectives and with much energy.

More specifically, we anticipate that our increasing understanding of the interpersonal contexts of aging will lead to further refinements in the construct of relational competence, and in our two-component model in particular. Future studies of relational competence in very old age, for example, may permit a greater understanding of the enhancement component of the model, its role in stabilizing high-dependency relationships, and its importance relative to the initiation component of the model. Similarly, a longitudinal study of relational competence may clarify how it impacts development of family systems, health, self-image, and those other, unique factors that determine the experience of old age.

References

Adelman, R. D., Greene, M. G., & Charon, R. (1987). The physician–elderly patient–companion triad in the medical encounter: The development of a conceptual framework and research agenda. *The Gerontologist, 27,* 729–734.

Adler, A. (1930). Individual psychology. In C. Murchison (Ed.), *Psychologies of 1930* (pp. 395–405). Worcester, MA: Clark University Press.

Aldwin, C. M. (1990). The elders life stress inventory: Egocentric and nonegocentric stress. In M. A. P. Stephens, J. H. Crowther, S. E. Hobfoll, & D. L. Tennenbaum (Eds.), *Stress and coping in later-life families* (pp. 49–69). New York: Hemisphere.

Alexander, G., & Lewin, T. (1972). *The aged and the need for surrogate management.* Syracuse, NY: Syracuse University Press.

Allen, G. A., & Adams, R. G. (1989). Aging and the structure of friendship. In R. G. Adams & R. Blieszner (Eds.), *Older adult friendship: Structure and process* (pp. 45–64). Newbury Park, CA: Sage.

American Association of Retired Persons. (1990). *A profile of older Americans: 1990.* Washington, DC: Author.

American Psychiatric Association. (1987). *Diagnostic and statistical manual of mental disorders* (3rd ed., revised) (DSM-III-R). Washington, DC: Author.

Antonucci, T. C. (1985). Personal characteristics, social support, and social behavior. In R. H. Binstock & E. Shanas (Eds.), *Handbook of aging and the social sciences* (2nd ed., pp. 94–128). New York: Van Nostrand Reinhold.

Antonucci, T., & Akiyama, H. (1987). Social networks in adult life and a preliminary examination of the convoy model. *Journal of Gerontology, 42,* 519–527.

Antonucci, T. C., & Jackson, J. S. (1987). Social support, interpersonal efficacy, and health: A life course perspective. In L. L. Carstensen & B. A. Edelstein (Eds.), *Handbook of clinical gerontology* (pp. 291–311). New York: Pergamon.

Arling, G., Harkins, E., & Capitman, J. (1986). Institutionalization and personal control. *Research on Aging, 8,* 38–56.

Atkins, C. J., Kaplan, R. M., & Toshima, M. T. (1991). Close relationships in the epidemiology of cardiovascular disease. In W. H. Jones & D. Perlman (Eds.), *Advances in personal relationships* (Vol. 3, pp. 207–231). London: Jessica Kingsley.

Auslander, G. K., & Litwin, H. (1990). Social support networks and formal help seeking: Differences between applicants to social services and a nonapplicant sample. *Journal of Gerontology: Social Sciences, 45,* S112–S119.

Bailey, L., & Hansson, R. O. (1993, November). *Age-related risks in job change among older workers.* Paper presented at the meeting of the Gerontological Society of America, New Orleans, LA.

Baltes, P. B. (1987). Theoretical propositions of life-span developmental psychology: On the dynamics between growth and decline. *Developmental Psychology, 23,* 611–626.

Baltes, P. B., & Baltes, M. M. (1990). Psychological perspectives on successful aging: The model of selective optimization with compensation. In P. B. Baltes & M. M. Baltes (Eds.), *Successful aging: Perspectives from the behavioral sciences* (pp. 1–34). Cambridge, England: Cambridge University Press.

Baltes, P. B., Reese, H. W., & Lipsitt, L. P. (1980). Life-span developmental psychology. *Annual Review of Psychology, 31,* 65–110.

Baltes, P. B., & Smith, J. (1990). Toward a psychology of wisdom and its ontogenesis. In R. J. Sternberg (Ed.), *Wisdom: Its nature, origins, and development* (pp. 87–120). New York: Cambridge University Press.

Bandura, A. (1977). Self-efficacy: Toward a unifying theory of behavioral change. *Psychological Review, 84,* 191–215.

Barefoot, J. C., Siegler, J. C., Nowlin, J. B., Peterson, B. L., Haney, T. L., & Williams, R. B. (1987). Suspiciousness, health, and mortality: A follow-up study of 500 older adults. *Psychosomatic Medicine, 49,* 450–457.

Barrera, M., & Baca, L. M. (1990). Recipient reactions to social support: Contributions of enacted support, conflicted support and network orientation. *Journal of Social and Personal Relationships, 7,* 541–551.

Barta Kvitek, S. D., Shaver, B. J., Blood, H., & Shepard, K. F. (1986). Age bias: Physical therapists and older patients. *Journal of Gerontology, 41,* 706–709.

Barusch, A. S. (1988). Problems and coping strategies of elderly spouse caregivers. *The Gerontologist, 28,* 677–685.

Bass, D. M., & Noelker, L. S. (1987). The influence of family caregivers on elder's use of in-home services: An expanded conceptual framework. *Journal of Health and Social Behavior, 28,* 184–196.

Bayles, F., & McCartney, S. (1987, September 20). Tangled guardianship system mistreats nation's elderly. *Tulsa World,* p. A-5.

Bear, M. (1990). Social network characteristics and the duration of primary relationships after entry into long-term care. *Journal of Gerontology: Social Sciences, 45,* S156–S162.

Bellack, S. A., & Hersen, M. (1977). *Behavior modification: An introductory textbook.* Baltimore: Williams & Wilkins.

Berkman, L. (1985). The relationship of social networks and social support to morbidity and mortality. In S. Cohen & S. L. Syme (Eds.), *Social support and health* (pp. 241–262). New York: Academic Press.

Berkman, L. F., & Breslow, L. (1983). *Health and ways of living: Findings from the Alameda County study.* New York: Oxford University Press.

Berman, S., Delaney, N., Gallagher, D., Atkins, P., & Graeber, M. P. (1987). Respite care: A partnership between a Veterans Administration nursing home and families to care for frail elders at home. *The Gerontologist, 27,* 581–584.

Bierman, R. (1969). Dimensions of interpersonal facilitation in psychotherapy and child development. *Psychological Bulletin, 72,* 338–352.

Bitzan, J. E., & Kruzich, J. M. (1990). Interpersonal relationships of nursing home residents. *The Gerontologist, 30,* 385–390.

Blazer, D. G., Burchett, B., Service, C., & George, L. K. (1991). The association of age and depression among the elderly: An epidemiologic exploration. *Journal of Gerontology: Medical Sciences, 46,* M210–M215.

Blazer, D., Hughes, D. C., & George, L. K. (1987). The epidemiology of depression in an elderly community population. *The Gerontologist, 27,* 281–287.

Blieszner, R. (1989). Developmental processes of friendship. In R. G. Adams & R. Blieszner (Eds.), *Older adult friendship: Structure and process* (pp. 108–126). Newbury Park, CA: Sage.

Bowlby, J. (1969). *Attachment and loss, Vol. I. Attachment.* New York: Basic Books.

Bowlby, J. (1973). *Attachment and loss, Vol. II. Separation: Anxiety and anger.* New York: Basic Books.

Bowlby, J. (1980). *Attachment and loss, Vol. III. Loss: Sadness and depression.* New York: Basic Books.

Brandtstadter, J., & Renner, G. (1990). Tenacious goal pursuit and flexible goal adjustment: Explication and age-related analysis of assimilative and accommodative strategies of coping. *Psychology and Aging, 5,* 58–67.

Brody, E. M. (1985). Parent care as a normative family stress. *The Gerontologist, 25,* 19–29.

Bulcroft, K., Kielkopf, M. R., & Tripp, K. (1991). Elderly wards and their legal guardians: Analysis of county probate records in Ohio and Washington. *The Gerontologist, 31,* 156–164.

Burns, G. L., & Farina, A. (1984). Social competence and adjustment. *Journal of Social and Personal Relationships, 1,* 99–113.

Busse, E. W. (1987). Mental health. In G. L. Maddox (Ed.), *The encyclopedia of aging* (pp. 438–439). New York: Springer.

Butler, R. N. (1975). *Why survive? Being old in America.* New York: Harper & Row.

Cantor, M. H. (1979). Neighbors and friends: An overlooked resource in the informal support system. *Research on Aging, 1,* 434–463.

Cantor, M. H. (1983). Strain among caregivers: A study of experience in the United States. *The Gerontologist, 23,* 597–604.

Cantor, M. H. (1991). Family and community: Changing roles in an aging society. *The Gerontologist, 31,* 337–346.

Cantor, M. H., & Little, V. (1985). Aging and social care. In R. H. Binstock & E. Shanas (Eds.), *Handbook of aging and the social sciences* (2nd ed., pp. 745–781). New York: Van Nostrand Reinhold.

Cappeliez, P. (1988). Some thoughts on the prevalence and etiology of depressive conditions in the elderly. *Canadian Journal on Aging, 7,* 431–440.

Carlo, G., Eisenberg, N., Troyer, D., Switzer, G., & Speer, A. L. (1991). The altruistic personality: In what contexts is it apparent? *Journal of Personality and Social Psychology, 61,* 450–458.

Carpenter, B. N. (1985, August). *Disentangling effects of stress, social support, and personality on functioning.* Paper presented at the annual convention of the American Psychological Association, Los Angeles, CA.

Carpenter, B. N. (1987, August). *Development, structure, and concurrent validity of the Relational Competence Scale.* Paper presented at the annual convention of the American Psychological Association, New York, NY.

Carpenter, B. N. (1993a). Relational competence. In D. Perlman & W. H. Jones (Eds.), *Advances in personal relationships* (Vol. 4, pp. 1–28). New York: Jessica Kingsley.

Carpenter, B. N. (1993b). *Relationships, relational competence, and relocation adjustment.* Unpublished manuscript, University of Tulsa.

Carpenter, B. N., & Scott, S. M. (1990, June). *Dimensions of stress situations.* Paper presented at the annual convention of the American Psychological Society, Dallas, TX.

Carpenter, B. N., & Scott, S. M. (1992). Interpersonal aspects of coping. In B. N. Carpenter (Ed.), *Personal coping: Theory, research, and application* (pp. 93–109). New York: Praeger.

Carpenter, B. N., & Suhr, P. (1988, August). *Stress appraisal: Measurement and correlates.* Paper presented at the annual meeting of the American Psychological Association, Atlanta, GA.

Carpenter, B. N., Hansson, R. O., Rountree, R., & Jones, W. H. (1983). Relational competence and adjustment in diabetic patients. *Journal of Social and Clinical Psychology, 1,* 359–369.

Carson, R. C. (1969). *Interaction concepts of personality.* Chicago: Aldine.

Cheek, J. M., & Buss, A. H. (1981). Shyness and sociability. *Journal of Personality and Social Psychology, 41,* 330–339.

Cohen, G. D. (1990). Psychopathology and mental health in the mature and elderly adult. In J. E. Birren & K. W. Schaie (Eds.), *Handbook of the psychology of aging* (3rd ed., pp. 359–371). San Diego: Academic Press.

Cohen, S., & McKay, G. (1984). Social support, stress, and the buffering hypothesis: A theoretical analysis. In A. Baum, S. E. Taylor, & J. E. Singer (Eds.), *Handbook of psychology and health* (Vol. IV, pp. 253–367). Hillsdale, NJ: Lawrence Erlbaum.

Cohen, S., & Syme, S. L. (Eds.). (1985). *Social support and health.* New York: Academic Press.

Colby, B. N., Aldwin, C., Price, L., & Mishra, S. (1985). Adaptive potential, stress, and illness in the elderly. *Medical Anthropology, 94,* 283–296.

Conger, J. C., & Conger, A. J. (1982). Components of heterosocial competence. In J. P. Curran & P. M. Monti (Eds.), *Social skills training* (pp. 313–347). New York: Guilford Press.

Connidis, I. A., & Davies, L. (1992). Confidants and companions: Choices in later life. *Journal of Gerontology: Social Sciences, 47,* S115–S122.

Costa, P. T., Jr., & McCrae, R. R. (1985). *The NEO Personality Inventory manual.* Odessa, FL: Psychological Assessment Resources.

Costa, P. T., Jr., & McCrae, R. R. (1993). *Revised NEO Personality Inventory (NEO PI-R) and NEO Five-Factor Inventory (NEO-FFI): Professional manual.* Odessa, FL: Psychological Assessment Resources.

Costa, P. T., Jr., McCrae, R. R., & Norris, A. H. (1981). Personal adjustment to aging: Longitudinal prediction from neuroticism and extraversion. *Journal of Gerontology, 36,* 78–85.

Council on Scientific Affairs. (1987). Council report: Elder abuse and neglect. *Journal of the American Medical Association, 257,* 966–971.

Cox, E. O., & Parsons, R. J. (1992). Senior-to-senior mediation service project. *The Gerontologist, 32,* 420–422.

Curran, J. (1977). Skills training as an approach to the treatment of heterosexual-social anxiety: A review. *Psychological Bulletin, 84,* 140–157.

Cutrona, C. E. (1982). Transition to college: Loneliness and the process of social adjustment. In L. A. Peplau & D. Perlman (Eds.), *Loneliness: A sourcebook of current theory, research, and therapy* (pp. 291–309). New York: Wiley-Interscience.

Cutrona, C. E., & Russell, D. W. (1987). The provisions of social relationships and adaptation to stress. In W. H. Jones & D. Perlman (Eds.), *Advances in personal relationship* (Vol. 1, pp. 37–67). New York: JAI Press.

Daniels, R. S., Baumhover, L. A., & Clark-Daniels, C. L. (1989). Physicians' mandatory reporting of elder abuse. *The Gerontologist, 29,* 321–327.

Davis, L. V., & Hagen, J. L. (1992). The problem of wife abuse: The interrelationship of social policy and social work practice. *Social Work, 37,* 15–20.

Davis, M. H., & Oathout, H. A. (1987). Maintenance of satisfaction in romantic relationships: Empathy and relational competence. *Journal of Personality and Social Psychology, 53,* 397–410.

Davis, V. K., & Carpenter, B. N. (1987, April). *Relational competence and marital satisfaction.* Paper presented at the annual meeting of the Southwestern Psychological Association, New Orleans, LA.

Dean, A., Kology, B., Wood, P., & Matt, G. E. (1992). The influence of living alone on depression in elderly persons. *Journal of Aging and Health, 4,* 3–18.

Derlega, V. J., Hendrick, S. S., Winstead, B. A., Berg, J. H. (1991). *Psychotherapy as a personal relationship.* New York: Guilford Press.

Digman, J. M., & Inouye, J. (1986). Further specification of the five robust factors of personality. *Journal of Personality and Social Psychology, 50,* 116–123.

DiMatteo, M. R. (1991). *The psychology of health, illness, and medical care: An individual perspective.* Pacific Grove, CA: Brooks/Cole.

Doll, E. A. (1935). The measurement of social competence. *American Association on Mental Deficiency, 40,* 103–126.

Donaldson, J. E. (1991, July). The ethical considerations of representing the elderly. *Trusts & Estates,* pp. 18–27.

Dubbert, P. M., & Wilson, G. T. (1984). Goal-setting and spouse involvement in the treatment of obesity. *Behaviour Research and Therapy, 13,* 227–242.

Duck, S. W. (Ed.). (1988a). *Handbook of personal relationships*. Chichester, England: Wiley.

Duck, S. (1988b). *Relating to others*. Chicago: Dorsey Press.

Dura, J. R., Stukenberg, K. W., & Kiecolt-Glaser, J. K. (1991). Anxiety and depressive disorders in adult children caring for demented parents. *Psychology and Aging, 6,* 467–473.

Dykman, B., & Reis, H. T. (1979). Personality correlates of classroom seating position. *Journal of Educational Psychology, 71,* 346–354.

Ekerdt, D. J. (1989). Retirement preparation. In M. P. Lawton (Ed.), *Annual review of gerontology and geriatrics* (Vol. 9, pp. 321–356). New York: Springer.

Engels, M. L. (1991). The promotion of positive social interaction through social skills training. In P. A. Wisocki (Ed.), *Handbook of clinical behavior therapy with the elderly client: Applied clinical psychology* (pp. 185–202). New York: Plenum Press.

Epstein, S. (1980). The stability of behavior: I. On predicting most of the people much of the time. *Journal of Personality and Social Psychology, 37,* 1097–1126.

Eustis, N. N., & Fischer, L. R. (1991). Relationships between home care clients and their workers: Implications for quality of care. *The Gerontologist, 31,* 447–456.

Eyde, D. R., & Rich, J. A. (1983). *Psychological stress in aging*. Rockville, MD: Aspen.

Eysenck, H. J. (1992). Four ways five factors are not basic. *Personality and Individual Differences, 13,* 667–673.

Feller, I., Flora, J. D. Jr., & Bawol, R. (1976). Baseline results of therapy for burned patients. *Journal of the American Medical Association, 236,* 1943–1947.

Felton, B. J. (1990). Coping and social support in older people's experiences of chronic illness. In M. A. P. Stephens, J. H. Crowther, S. E. Hobfoll, & D. L. Tennenbaum (Eds.), *Stress and coping in later-life families* (pp. 153–171). New York: Hemisphere.

Finley, G. E. (1982). Modernization and aging. In T. M. Field, A. Huston, H. C. Quay, L. Troll, & G. E. Finley (Eds.), *Review of human development* (pp. 511–523). New York: Wiley-Interscience.

Fisher, G., & Tessler, R. (1986). Family bonding of the mentally ill: An analysis of family visits with residents of board and care homes. *Journal of Health and Social Behavior, 27,* 236–249.

Fletcher, W. L., & Hansson, R. O. (1991). Assessing the social components of retirement anxiety. *Psychology and Aging, 6,* 76–85.

Folkman, S., Lazarus, R. S., Pimley, S., & Novacek, J. (1987). Age differences in stress and coping processes. *Psychology and Aging, 2,* 171–184.

Franzke, A. W. (1987). The effects of assertiveness training on older adults. *The Gerontologist, 27,* 13–16.

Fredriksen, K. I. (1992). North of Market: Older Women's Alcohol Outreach Program. *The Gerontologist, 32,* 270–272.

Freedberg, S. P. (1987, October 13). Forced exits? Companies confront wave of age-discrimination suits. *Wall Street Journal,* p. 37.

Freud, S. (1957). Mourning and melancholia. In J. Stachey (Ed.), *The standard edition of the complete psychological works of Sigmund Freud* (Vol. 14). London: Hogarth. (Original work published 1917)

Friedman, H. S., & Booth-Kewley, S. (1987). The "disease-prone personality": A meta-analytic view of the construct. *American Psychologist, 42, 539–555.*

Friedman, M., & Rosenman, R. H. (1974). *Type A behavior and your heart.* New York: Knopf.

Fry, P. S. (1986). *Depression, stress, and adaptations in the elderly: Psychological assessment and intervention.* Rockville, MD: Aspen.

Funder, D. C., & Dobroth, K. M. (1987). Differences between traits: Properties associated with interjudge agreement. *Journal of Personality and Social Psychology, 52, 409–418.*

Gable, S., Belsky, J., & Crnic, K. (1992). Marriage, parenting, and child development: Progress and prospects. *Journal of Family Psychology, 5, 276–294.*

Gallagher-Thompson, D., Futterman, A., Farberow, N., Thompson, L. W., & Peterson, J. (1993). The impact of spousal bereavement on older widows and widowers. In M. Stroebe, W. Stroebe, and R. O. Hansson (Eds.), *The handbook of bereavement* (pp. 227–239). New York: Cambridge University Press.

Garcia, S., Stinson, L., Ickes, W., Bissonnette, V., & Briggs, S. R. (1991). Shyness and physical attractiveness in mixed-sex dyads. *Journal of Personality and Social Psychology, 61, 35–49.*

Garfield, S. L., & Bergin, A. E. (Eds.). (1987). *Handbook of psychotherapy and behavior change* (3rd ed.). New York: Wiley.

Gatz, M. (1988, August). *Clinical psychology and aging.* Master lecture delivered at the annual convention of the American Psychological Association, Atlanta, GA.

Gatz, M., Bengtson, V. L., & Blum, M. J. (1990). Caregiving families. In J. E. Birren & K. W. Schaie (Eds.), *Handbook of the psychology of aging* (3rd ed., pp. 404–425). San Diego: Academic Press.

Gatz, M., Popkin, S. J., Pino, C. D., & VandenBos, G. R. (1985). Psychological interventions with older adults. In J. E. Birren & K. W. Schaie (Eds.), *Handbook of the psychology of aging* (2nd ed, pp. 755–785). New York: Van Nostrand Reinhold.

Gatz, M., & Smyer, M. A. (1992). The mental health system and older adults in the 1990s. *American Psychologist, 47, 741–751.*

Gaylord, S. A., & Zung, W. W. K. (1987). Affective disorders among the aging. In L. L. Carstensen & B. A. Edelstein (Eds.), *Handbook of clinical gerontology* (pp. 76–95). New York: Pergamon.

George, L. (1988). Social participation in later life: Black–white differences. In J. S. Jackson (Ed.), *The black American elderly* (pp. 99–126). New York: Springer.

George, L. K. (1987). Non-familial support for older persons: Who is out there and how can they be reached? In G. Lesnoff-Caravaglia (Ed.), *Handbook of applied gerontology* (pp. 310–322). New York: Human Sciences Press.

George, L. K., & Gwyther, L. P. (1986). Caregiver well-being: A multidimensional examination of family caregivers and demented adults. *The Gerontologist, 2,* 253–259.

Gold, P. W., Goodwin, F. K., & Chrousos, G. P. (1988). Clinical and biochemical manifestations of depression: Relation to the neurobiology of stress (second of two parts). *New England Journal of Medicine, 319,* 413–420.

Goldberg, L. R. (1992). The development of markers for the big-five factor structure. *Psychological Assessment, 4,* 26–42.

Goldberg, L. R. (1993). The structure of phenotypic personality traits. *American Psychologist, 48,* 26–34.

Goodman, C. C., & Pynoos, J. (1988). Telephone networks connect caregiving families of Alzheimer's victims. *The Gerontologist, 5,* 602–605.

Graham, J. R., & Strenger, V. E. (1988). MMPI characteristics of alcoholics: A review. *Journal of Consulting and Clinical Psychology, 56,* 197–205.

Greene, V., & Monahan, D. (1982). The impact of visitation on patient well-being in nursing homes. *The Gerontologist, 22,* 418–423.

Greene, V. L., & Monahan, D. J. (1987). The effect of a professionally guided caregiver support and education group on institutionalization of care receivers. *The Gerontologist, 27,* 716–721.

Guberman, N., Maheu, P., & Maille, C. (1992). Women as family caregivers: Why do they care? *The Gerontologist, 32,* 607–617.

Gurian, B. S. (1992). Transportation as outreach, driver as mental health worker. *The Gerontologist, 32,* 561–562.

Gurtman, M. B. (1992). Trust, distrust, and interpersonal problems: A circumplex analysis. *Journal of Personality and Social Psychology, 62,* 989–1002.

Hagedorn, A. (1990, June 25). States lack funds to deal with rising elder abuse. *Wall Street Journal,* p. B-1.

Halpert, B. P. (1988). Volunteer information provider program: A strategy to reach and help rural family caregivers. *The Gerontologist, 28,* 256–259.

Hansson, R. O. (1986a). Relational competence, relationships, and adjustment in old age. *Journal of Personality and Social Psychology, 50,* 1050–1058.

Hansson, R. O. (1986b). Shyness and the elderly. In W. H. Jones, J. M. Cheek, & S. R. Briggs (Eds.), *Shyness: Perspectives on research and treatment* (pp. 117–129). New York: Plenum Press.

Hansson, R. O., Briggs, S. R., & Rule, B. L. (1990). Old age and unemployment: Predictors of perceived control, depression, and loneliness. *Journal of Applied Gerontology, 9,* 230–240.

Hansson, R. O., & Carpenter, B. N. (1986). Coping with fear of crime among the elderly. *Clinical Gerontologist, 4,* 38–40.

Hansson, R. O., & Carpenter, B. N. (1990). Relational competence and adjustment in older adults: Implications for the demands of aging. In M.

A. P. Stephens, J. H. Crowther, S. E. Hobfoll, & D. L. Tennenbaum (Eds.), *Stress and coping in later life families* (pp. 131–151). Washington, DC: Hemisphere.

Hansson, R. O., Fairchild, S., Vanzetti, N., & Harris, G. (1992, July). *The nature of family bereavement.* Paper presented at the International Conference on Personal Relationships, Orono, ME.

Hansson, R. O., Hogan, R., Johnson, J. A., & Schroeder, D. (1983). Disentangling Type A behavior: The roles of ambition, insensitivity, and anxiety. *Journal of Research in Personality, 17,* 186–197.

Hansson, R. O., Jones, W. H., & Carpenter, B. N. (1984). Relational competence and social support. In P. Shaver (Ed.), *Review of personality and social psychology: Vol. 5. Emotions, relationships, and health* (pp. 265–284). Beverly Hills: Sage.

Hansson, R. O., Jones, W. H., Carpenter, B. N., & Remondet, J. H. (1986). Loneliness and adjustment to old age. *International Journal of Aging and Human Development, 24,* 41–53.

Hansson, R. O., Jones, W. H., & Fletcher, W. F. (1990). Troubled relationships in later life: Implications for support. *Journal of Social and Personal Relationships, 7,* 451–463.

Hansson, R. O., Nelson, R. E., Carver, M. D., NeeSmith, D. H., Dowling, E. M., Fletcher, W. L., & Suhr, P. (1990). Adult children with frail elderly parents: When to intervene? *Family Relations, 39,* 153–158.

Hansson, R. O., Remondet, J. H., & Galusha, M. (1993). Old age and widowhood: Issues of personal control and independence. In M. S. Stroebe, W. Stroebe, & R. O. Hansson, (Eds.), *Handbook of bereavement: Theory, research, and intervention* (pp. 367–380). Cambridge, England: Cambridge University Press.

Hansson, R. O., Remondet, J. H., Obrochta, D., & Bell, L. (1988). The dissatisfied medical patient: Predictors of intent to change doctors. *Medical Times, 116*(12), 97–101.

Hansson, R. O., Slade, K. M., Nelson, S. A., Carpenter, B. N., & Rountree, R. (1983). *Social assertiveness among permanently disabled, diabetic, and older adults.* Paper presented at the annual meeting of the American Psychological Association, Anaheim, CA.

Harel, Z., & Noelker, L. (1982). Social integration, health, and choice: Their impact on the well-being of institutionalized aged. *Research on Aging, 4,* 97–111.

Hayslip, B., Jr., & Leon, J. (1992). *Hospice care.* Newbury Park, CA: Sage.

Heath, G. W., Hagberg, J. M., Ehsani, A. A., & Holloszy, J. O. (1981). A physiological comparison of young and older endurance athletes. *Journal of Applied Physiology, 51,* 634–640.

Heiselman, T., & Noelker, L. S. (1991). Enhancing mutual respect among nursing assistants, residents, and residents' families. *The Gerontologist, 31,* 552–555.

Heller, K., Thompson, M. G., Trueba, P. E., Hogg, J. R., & Vlachos-Weber, I. (1991). Peer support telephone dyads for elderly women: Was this the wrong intervention? *American Journal of Community Psychology, 19,* 53–74.

Hickey, T. (1980). *Health and aging.* Monterey, CA: Brooks/Cole.

Hinrichsen, G. A. (1991). Adjustment of caregivers to depressed older adults. *Psychology and Aging, 6,* 631–639.

Hobfoll, S. (1992, August). *The Strategic Approach to Coping Scale.* Paper presented at the annual convention of the American Psychological Association, Washington, DC.

Hobfoll, S. E. (1988). *The ecology of stress.* New York: Hemisphere.

Hogan, R., & Hogan, J. (1992). *Hogan Personality Inventory manual.* Tulsa, OK: Hogan Assessment Systems.

Hogg, J. R., & Heller, K. (1990). A measure of relational competence for community-dwelling elderly. *Psychology and Aging, 5,* 580–588.

Hogstel, M. O., & Gaul, A. L. (1991). Safety or autonomy. *Journal of Gerontological Nursing, 17,* 6–11.

Horowitz, A. (1985). Family caregiving to the frail elderly. *Annual review of gerontology and geriatrics, 5,* 194–246.

Horowitz, A., & Shindelman, L. (1983). Reciprocity and affection: Past influences on current caregiving. *Journal of Gerontological Social Work, 5,* 5–19.

Horowitz, L. M., & Vitkus, J. (1986). The interpersonal basis of psychiatric symptoms. *Clinical Psychology Review, 6,* 443–469.

Horowitz, M. J., Marmar, C., Weiss, D. S., DeWitt, K. N., & Rosenbaum, R. (1984). Brief psychotherapy of grief reactions. *Archives of General Psychiatry, 41,* 439–448.

House, J. S. (1981). *Work, stress and social support.* Reading, MA: Addison-Wesley.

House, J. S., Landis, K. R., & Umberson, D. (1988). Social relationships and health. *Science, 241,* 540–545.

Institute of Medicine. (1986). *Improving the quality of care in nursing homes.* Washington, DC: National Academy Press.

Iris, M. (1988). Guardianship and the elderly: A multi-perspective view of the decision making process. *The Gerontologist, 28*(Suppl.), 39–45.

Irwin, M., & Pike, J. (1993). Bereavement, depressive symptoms, and immune function. In M. S. Stroebe, W. Stroebe, & R. O. Hansson (Eds.), *Handbook of bereavement: Theory, research, and intervention* (pp. 160–171). Cambridge, England: Cambridge University Press.

Jackson, D. N. (1970). A sequential system for personality scale development. In C. D. Spielberger (Ed.), *Current topics in clinical and community psychology* (pp. 61–96). New York: Academic Press.

Johnson, C. L. (1983). Dyadic family relations and social support. *The Gerontologist, 23,* 377–383.

Johnson, C. L., & Barer, B. M. (1990). Families and networks among older inner-city blacks. *The Gerontologist, 30,* 726–733.

Johnson, C. L., & Catalano, D. J. (1983). A longitudinal study of family supports to impaired elderly. *The Gerontologist, 23,* 612–618.

Jones, D. C., & Vaughan, K. (1990). Close friendships among senior adults. *Psychology and Aging, 5,* 451–457.

Jones, W. H. (1985). The psychology of loneliness: Some personality issues in the study of social support. In I. G. Sarason & B. R. Sarason (Eds.), *Social support: Theory, research and application* (pp. 225–241). Dordrecht, The Netherlands: Martinus Nijhoff.

Jones, W. H., & Briggs, S. R. (1984). The self-other discrepancy in social shyness. In R. Schwarzer (Ed.), *The self in anxiety, stress and depression* (pp. 93–107). Amsterdam: North Holland.

Jones, W. H., & Briggs, S. R. (1986). *Manual for the Social Reticence Scale (SRS): A measure of shyness.* Palo Alto, CA: Consulting Psychologists Press.

Jones, W. H., & Carpenter, B. N. (1986). Shyness, social behavior, and relationships. In W. H. Jones, J. M. Cheek, & S. R. Briggs (Eds.), *Shyness: Perspectives on research and treatment* (pp. 227–238). New York: Plenum Press.

Jones, W. H., Carpenter, B. N., & Quintana, D. (1985). Personality and interpersonal predictors of loneliness in two cultures. *Journal of Personality and Social Psychology, 48,* 1503–1511.

Jones, W. H., Cavert, C., & Indart, M. (1983, August). *Impressions of shyness.* Paper presented at the annual meeting of the American Psychological Association, Anaheim, CA.

Jones, W. H., Hobbs, S., & Hockenbury, D. (1982). Loneliness and social skill deficits. *Journal of Personality and Social Psychology, 42,* 682–689.

Jones, W. H., & Russell, D. (1982). The social reticence scale: An objective instrument to measure shyness. *Journal of Personality Assessment, 46,* 629–631.

Kahn, R. L. (1975). The mental health system and the future aged. *The Gerontologist, 15,* 24–31.

Kahn, R. L., & Antonucci, T. C. (1980). Convoys over the life course: Attachment, roles and social support. In P. B. Baltes & O. G. Brim (Eds.), *Lifespan development and behavior.* New York: Academic Press.

Kamptner, N. L. (1989). Personal possessions and their meanings in old age. In S. Spacapan & S. Oskamp (Eds.), *The social psychology of aging* (pp. 165–196). Newbury Park, CA: Sage.

Kane, R. A., & Kane, R. L. (1981). *Assessing the elderly: A practical guide to measurement.* Lexington, MA: Lexington.

Kaplan, R. M., & Toshima, M. T. (1990). Social relationships in chronic illness and disability. In I. G. Sarason, B. R. Sarason, & G. R. Pierce (Eds.), *Social support: An interactional perspective* (pp. 427–453). New York: Wiley.

Kaplan, R. M., Sallis, J. F., Jr., & Patterson, T. L. (1993). *Health and human behavior.* New York: McGraw-Hill.

Katz, S., Branch, L. G., Branson, M. H., Papsidero, J. A., Beck, J. C., & Greer, D. S. (1983). Active life expectancy. *New England Journal of Medicine, 309,* 130–135.

Keith, P. M. (1987). Depressive symptoms among younger and older couples. *The Gerontologist, 27,* 605–610.

Kemp, B. (1985). Rehabilitation and the older adult. In J. E. Birren & K. W. Schaie (Eds.), *Handbook of the psychology of aging* (2nd ed., pp. 647–663). New York: Van Nostrand Reinhold.

Kiecolt-Glaser, J. K., Garner, W., Speicher, C., Penn, G., Holliday, E. S., &

Glaser, R. (1984). Psychosocial modifiers of immunocompetence in medical students. *Psychosomatic Medicine, 46*, 7–14.

Kiecolt-Glaser, J. K., Ricker, D., George, J., Messick, G., Speicher, C., Garner, W., & Glaser, R. (1984). Urinary cortisol levels, cellular immunocompetency, and loneliness in psychiatric inpatients. *Psychosomatic Medicine, 46*, 523–535.

Kingson, E. R., Hirshorn, B. A., & Cornman, J. M. (1986). *Ties that bind: The interdependence of generations.* Washington, DC: Seven Locks Press.

Kirkpatrick, R. V., & Patchner, M. A. (1987). The utilization of peer counselors for the provision of mental health services to the aged. *Clinical Gerontologist, 6*(4), 3–14.

Knight, B. G., Lutzky, S. M., & Macofsky-Urban, F. (1993). A meta-analytic review of interventions for caregiver distress: Recommendations for future research. *The Gerontologist, 33,* 240–248.

Kobasa, S. C. (1979). Stressful life events, personality and health: An inquiry into hardiness. *Journal of Personality and Social Psychology, 37,* 1–11.

Korte, C., & Gupta, V. (1991). A program of friendly visitors as network builders. *The Gerontologist, 31*, 404–407.

Kosberg, J. I. (1988). Preventing elder abuse: Identification of high risk factors prior to placement decisions. *The Gerontologist, 28*, 43–50.

Kosberg, J. I., & Cairl, R. E. (1986). The cost of care index: A case management tool for screening informal care providers. *The Gerontologist, 26*, 273–278.

Krause, N. (1987). Chronic financial strain, social support, and depressive symptoms among older adults. *Psychology and Aging, 2*, 185–192.

Krause, N. (1991). Stress and isolation from close ties in later life. *Journal of Gerontology: Social Sciences, 46*, S183–S194.

Labouvie-Vief, G. (1985). Intelligence and cognition. In J. E. Birren & K. W. Schaie (Eds.), *Handbook of the psychology of aging* (2nd ed., pp. 500–530). New York: Van Nostrand Reinhold.

la Gory, M., & Fitzpatrick, K. (1992). The effects of environmental context on elderly depression. *Journal of Aging and Health, 5*, 459–479.

Laudenslager, M. L. (1988). The psychobiology of loss: Lessons from humans and nonhuman primates. *Journal of Social Issues, 44*, 19–36.

Lawton, M. P. (1980). *Environment and aging.* Monterey, CA: Brooks/Cole.

Lawton, M. P. (1981). Community supports for the aged. *Journal of Social Issues, 37*, 102–115.

Lawton, M. P., & Hoover, S. (Eds.). (1981). *Community housing choices for older Americans.* New York: Springer.

Lawton, M. P., & Moss, M. (1987). The social relationships of older people. In E. F. Borgatta & R. J. V. Montgomery (Eds.), *Critical issues in aging policy: Linking research and values* (pp. 92–126). Newbury Park, CA: Sage.

Lawton, M. P., & Simon, B. B. (1968). The ecology of social relationships in housing for the elderly. *Gerontologist, 8*, 110–115.

Lazarus, R., & Folkman, S. (1984). *Stress, appraisal, and coping.* New York: Springer.

Leary, T. (1957). *Interpersonal diagnosis of personality*. New York: Ronald.

Lefcourt, H. M. (1991). Locus of control. In J. P. Robinson, P. R. Shaver, & L. S. Wrightsman (Eds.), *Measures of personality and social psychological attitudes* (pp. 413–499). San Diego: Academic Press.

Lefcourt, H. M. (1992). Perceived control, personal effectiveness, and emotional states. In B. N. Carpenter (Ed.), *Personal coping: Theory, research, and application* (pp. 111–131). New York: Praeger.

Lerner, M. J., Somers, D. G., Reid, D. W., & Tierney, M. C. (1989). A social dilemma: Egocentrically biased cognitions among filial caregivers. In S. Spacapan & S. Oskamp (Eds.), *The social psychology of aging* (pp. 53–80). Newbury Park, CA: Sage.

Levinson, D. J. (1986). A conception of adult development. *American Psychologist, 41,* 3–13.

Levinson, D. J., with Darrow, C. N., Klein, E. B., Livinson, M. H., & McKee, B. (1978). *The seasons of a man's life*. New York: Knopf.

Libet, J. M., & Lewinsohn, P. M. (1973). Concept of social skill with special reference to the behavior of depressed persons. *Journal of Consulting and Clinical Psychology, 40,* 304–312.

Lieberman, M. A. (1983). Comparative analyses of change mechanisms in groups. In H. H. Blumberg, A. P. Hare, V. Kent, & M. Davies (Eds.), *Small groups and social interaction* (Vol. 2, pp. 239–252). New York: Wiley.

Lieberman, M. A. (1987). Self-help groups and the elderly: An overview. In E. E. Lurie & J. H. Swann (Eds.), *Serving the mentally ill elderly: Problems and perspectives* (pp. 163–176). Lexington, MA: Lexington Books.

Lieberman, M. A., & Videka-Sherman, L. (1986). The impact of self-help groups on the mental health of widows and widowers. *American Journal of Orthopsychiatry, 56,* 435–449.

Lopata, H. Z. (Ed.). (1987). *Widows: The Middle East, Asia and the Pacific* (Vol. 1). Durham, NC: Duke University Press.

Lopata, H. Z. (1988). Support systems of American urban widowhood. *Journal of Social Issues, 44,* 113–128.

Lund, D. A. (1989). *Older bereaved spouses: Research with practical applications*. New York: Hemisphere.

Lund, D. A., Caserta, M. S., & Dimond, M. F. (1993). The course of spousal bereavement in later life. In M. Stroebe, W. Stroebe, & R. Hansson (Eds.). *The handbook of bereavement* (pp. 240–254). New York: Cambridge University Press.

McCrae, R. R., & Costa, P. T., Jr. (1985). Updating Norman's "Adequate Taxonomy": Intelligence and personality dimensions in natural language and in questionnaires. *Journal of Personality and Social Psychology, 49,* 710–721.

McCrae, R. R., & Costa, P. T., Jr. (1989). The structure of interpersonal traits: Wiggins' circumplex and the five factor model. *Journal of Personality and Social Psychology, 56,* 586–595.

McFall, R. M. (1982). A review and reformulation of the concept of social skills. *Behavioral Assessment, 4,* 1–33.

McGovern, L. P. (1976). Dispositional social anxiety and helping behavior under three conditions of threat. *Journal of Personality, 44,* 84–97.

Meyerhoff, B. (1978). *Number our days.* New York: Simon & Schuster.

Mischel, W. (1973). Toward a cognitive social learning reconceptualization of personality. *Psychological Review, 80,* 252–283.

Mitchell, J., & Register, J. C. (1984). An exploration of family interaction with the elderly by race, socioeconomic status and residence. *The Gerontologist, 24,* 48–54.

Mohide, E. A., Pringle, D. M., Streiner, D. L., Gilbert, J. R., Muir, G., & Tew, M. (1990). A randomized trial of family caregiver support in the home management of dementia. *Journal of the American Geriatrics Society, 38,* 446–454.

Monroe, P. R. (1990). *A study of marital problems, marital satisfaction, and commitment.* Unpublished doctoral dissertation, The University of Tulsa.

Mor-Barak, M. E., Miller, L. S., & Syme, L. S. (1991). Social networks, life events, and health of the poor, frail elderly: A longitudinal study of the buffering versus the direct effect. *Family & Community Health, 14*(2), 1–13.

Morgan, D. L. (1982). Failing health and the desire for independence: Two conflicting aspects of health care in old age. *Social problems, 30,* 40–50.

Morgan, D. L. (1985). Nurses' perceptions of mental confusion in the elderly: Influence of resident and setting characteristics. *Journal of Health and Social Behavior, 26,* 102–112.

Morgan, T. J., Hansson, R. O., Indart, M. J., Austin, D. M., Crutcher, M., Hampton, P. W., Oppegard, K.M., & O'Daffer, V. E. (1984). Old age and environmental docility: The roles of health, support, and personality. *Journal of Gerontology, 39,* 240–242.

Morrison, J., & Hansson, R. O. (1993). *The social components of retirement anxiety: Personality predictors.* Unpublished manuscript, University of Tulsa.

Morrow-Howell, N., & Ozawa, M. N. (1987). Helping network: Seniors to seniors. *The Gerontologist, 27,* 17–20.

Mosak, H. H. (1989). Adlerian psychotherapy. In R. J. Corsini & D. Wedding (Ed.), *Current psychotherapies* (4th ed., pp. 65–116). Itasca, IL: F. E. Peacock.

Moss, M. S., & Pfohl, D. C. (1988). New friendships: Staff as visitors of nursing home residents. *The Gerontologist, 28,* 263–265.

Natale, M., Entin, E., & Jaffee, J. (1979). Vocal interruptions in dyadic communications as a function of speech and social anxiety. *Journal of Personality and Social Psychology, 37,* 865–878.

National Institute on Aging. (1978). *The older woman: Continuities and discontinuities.* NIH Publication No. 80-1897. Bethesda, MD: U.S. Department of Health and Human Services.

Neugarten, B. L., & Neugarten, D. A. (1986). Age in the aging society. *Daedalus, 115,* 31–49.

Nicholson, R. A., & Kugler, K. E. (1992). Competent and incompetent criminal defendants: A quantitative review of comparative research. *Psychological Bulletin, 109,* 355–370.

Norris, V. K., Stephens, M. A. P., & Kinney, J. M. (1990). The impact of family interactions on recovery from stroke: Help or hindrance? *The Gerontologist, 30,* 535–542.

Nuttbrock, L., & Kosberg, J. I. (1980). Images of the physician and help-seeking behavior of the elderly: A multivariate assessment. *Journal of Gerontology, 35,* 241–248.

O'Bryant, S. L., & Hansson, R. O. (In press). Widowhood. In R. Blieszner & V. Bedford (Eds.), *Handbook of aging and the family.* Westport, CT: Greenwood Press.

Ong, Y., Martineau, F., Lloyd, C., & Robbins, I. (1987). A support group for the depressed elderly. *International Journal of Geriatric Psychiatry, 2,* 119–123.

Osterweis, M., Solomon, F., & Green, M. (1984). *Bereavement: Reactions, consequences, and care.* Washington, DC: National Academy Press.

Parkes, C. M., & Weiss, R. S. (1983). *Recovery from bereavement.* New York: Basic Books.

Parmelee, P. A., Katz, I. R., & Lawton, M. P. (1992). Incidence of depression in long-term care settings. *Journal of Gerontology: Medical Sciences, 47,* M189–M196.

Parmelee, P. A., & Lawton, M. P. (1990). The design of special environments for the aged. In J. E. Birren & K. W. Schaie (Eds.), *Handbook of the psychology of aging* (3rd ed., pp. 464–488). San Diego: Academic Press.

Pearlin, L. I., Mullan, J. T., Semple, S. J., & Skaff, M. M. (1990). Caregiving and the stress process: An overview of concepts and their measures. *The Gerontologist, 30,* 583–594.

Pearlin, L. I., & Schooler, C. (1978). The structure of coping. *Journal of Health and Social Behavior, 19,* 2–22.

Pearlman, D. N., & Crown, W. H. (1992). Alternative sources of social support and their impacts on institutional risk. *The Gerontologist, 32,* 527–535.

Penning, M., & Wasyliw, D. (1992). Homebound learning opportunities: Reaching out to older shut-ins and their caregivers. *The Gerontologist, 32,* 704–707.

Perry, E. M., & Hansson, R. O. (1991, April). *Predictions of organizational power and influence among older workers.* Paper presented at the annual convention of the Southwestern Psychological Association, New Orleans, LA.

Perry, E. M., & Hansson, R. O. (1992, November). *Successful aging in organizations: Insights from the eminent.* Paper presented at the annual convention of the Gerontological Society of America, Washington, DC.

Pfeiffer, E. (1977). Psychopathology and social pathology. In J. E. Birren & K. W. Schaie (Eds.), *Handbook of the psychology of aging* (pp. 650–671). New York: Van Nostrand Reinhold.

Phillips, E. L. (1978). *The social skills basis of psychopathology: Alternative to abnormal psychology and psychiatry.* New York: Grune & Stratton.

Pietrukowicz, M. E., & Johnson, M. M. S. (1991). Using life histories to individualize nursing home staff attitudes toward residents. *The Gerontologist, 31,* 102–106.

Pilkonis, P. A. (1977). The behavioral consequences of shyness. *Journal of Personality, 45,* 596–611.

Pillemer, K., & Finkelhor, D. (1988). The prevalence of elder abuse: A random sample survey. *The Gerontologist, 28,* 51–57.

Pillemer, K., & Moore, D. W. (1989). Abuse of patients in nursing homes: Findings from a survey of staff. *The Gerontologist, 29,* 314–320.

Pinkston, E. M., & Linsk, N. L. (1984). Behavioral family intervention with the impaired elderly. *The Gerontologist, 24,* 576–583.

Poulshock, S. W., & Deimling, G. T. (1984). Families caring for elders in residence: Issues in the measurement of burden. *Journal of Gerontology, 39,* 230–239.

Pruchno, R., & Kleban, M. H. (1993). Caring for an institutionalized parent: The role of coping strategies. *Psychology and Aging, 8,* 18–25.

Rathus, S. A. (1973). A 30-item schedule for assessing assertive behavior. *Behavior Therapy, 4,* 398–406.

Reid, W. J., & Crisafulli, A. (1990). Marital discord and child behavior problems: A meta-analysis. *Journal of Abnormal Child Psychology, 18,* 105–117.

Retsinas, J., & Garrity, P. (1985). Nursing home friendships. *The Gerontologist, 25,* 376–381.

Reynolds, P., & Kaplan, G. A. (1990). Social connections and risk for cancer: Prospective evidence from the Alameda County Study. *Behavioral Medicine, 16,* 101–110.

Roberto, K. A. (1992). Coping strategies of older women with hip fractures: Resources and outcomes. *Journal of Gerontology: Psychological Sciences, 47,* P21–P26.

Robinson, B. C. (1983). Validation of a caregiver strain index. *Journal of Gerontology, 38,* 344–348.

Robinson, K. M. (1988). A social skills training program for adult caregivers. *Advances in Nursing Science, 10,* 59–72.

Rook, K. S. (1984). The negative side of social interaction: Impact on psychological well-being. *Journal of Personality and Social Psychology, 46,* 1097–1108.

Rook, K. S. (1987). Reciprocity of social exchange and social satisfaction among older women. *Journal of Personality and Social Psychology, 62,* 145–154.

Rook, K. S. (1989). Strains in older adults' friendships. In R. G. Adams, & R. Blieszner (Eds.), *Older adult friendship* (pp. 166–194). Newbury Park: Sage.

Rook, K. S. (1990). Stressful aspects of older adults' social relationships: Current theory and research. In M. A. P. Stephens, J. H. Crowther, S. E. Hobfoll, & D. L. Tennenbaum (Eds.), *Stress and coping in later-life families* (pp. 173–192). New York: Hemisphere.

Rook, K. S., & Pietromonaco, P. (1987). Close relationships: Ties that heal or ties that bind? In W. H. Jones & D. Perlman (Eds.), *Advances in personal relationships,* (Vol. 1, pp. 1–35). New York: JAI Press.

Rosenblatt, P. C. (1988). Grief: The social context of private feelings. *Journal of Social Issues, 44,* 67–78.

Rosenbloom, C. A., & Whittington, F. J. (1993). The effects of bereavement on eating behaviors and nutrient intakes in elderly widowed persons. *Journal of Gerontology: Social Sciences, 48,* S223–S229.

Rosow, I. (1985). Status and role change through the life cycle. In R. H. Binstock & E. Shanas (Eds.), *Handbook of aging and the social sciences* (2nd ed., pp. 62–93). New York: Van Nostrand Reinhold.

Rowe, J. W. (1977). Clinical research on aging: Strategies and directions. *New England Journal of Medicine, 297,* 1332–1336.

Rowe, J. W. (1985). Health care of the elderly. *New England Journal of Medicine, 312,* 827–835.

Rowe, J. W., & Kahn, R. L. (1987). Human aging: Usual and successful. *Science, 237,* 143–149.

Rowles, G. D. (1987). A place to call home. In L. L. Carstensen & B. A. Edelstein (Eds.), *Handbook of clinical gerontology* (pp. 335–353). New York: Pergamon.

Rubenstein, L. Z., Josephson, K. R., Nichol-Seamons, M., & Robbins, A. S. (1986). Comprehensive health screening of well elderly adults: An analysis of a community program. *Journal of Gerontology, 41,* 342–352.

Russell, D. W., & Cutrona, C. E. (1991). Social support, stress, and depressive symptoms among the elderly: Test of a process model. *Psychology and Aging, 6,* 190–201.

Russell, D., Peplau, L. A., & Cutrona, C. E. (1980). The Revised UCLA Loneliness Scale: Concurrent and discriminant validity evidence. *Journal of Personality and Social Psychology, 39,* 472–480.

Santee, R. T., & Maslach, C. (1982). To agree or not to agree: Personal dissent amid social pressure to conform. *Journal of Personality and Social Psychology, 42,* 690–700.

Sarason, B. R., Sarason, I. G., & Pierce, G. R. (Eds.). (1990). *Social support: An interactional view.* New York: Wiley.

Sayers, S. L., & Baucom, D. H. (1991). Role of femininity and masculinity in distressed couples' communication. *Journal of Personality and Social Psychology, 61,* 641–647.

Schaefer, C., Coyne, J. C., & Lazarus, R. S. (1981). The health-related functions of social support. *Journal of Behavioral Medicine, 4,* 381–406.

Schaie, K. W. (1983). The Seattle Longitudinal Study: A twenty-one year exploration of psychometric intelligence in adulthood. In K. W. Schaie (Ed.), *Longitudinal studies of adult psychological development* (pp. 64–135). New York: Guilford Press.

Schaie, K. W. (1990a). Intellectual development in adulthood. In J. E. Birren & K. W. Schaie (Eds.), *Handbook of the psychology of aging* (3rd ed., pp. 291–309). San Diego: Academic Press.

Schaie, K. W. (1990b). The optimization of cognitive functioning in old age: Predictions based on cohort-sequential and longitudinal data. In P. B. Baltes & M. M. Baltes (Eds.), *Successful aging: Perspectives from the behavioral sciences* (pp. 94–117). London: Cambridge University Press.

Schaie, K. W., & Willis, S. L. (1986). Can adult intellectual decline be reversed? *Developmental Psychology, 22,* 223–232.

Scharlach, A. E. (1988). Peer counselor training for nursing home residents. *The Gerontologist, 28,* 499–502.

Scharlach, A. E., & Boyd, S. L. (1989). Caregiving and employment: Results of an employee survey. *The Gerontologist, 29,* 382–387.

Schultz, R., Tompkins, C. A., & Rau, M. T. (1988). A longitudinal study of the psychosocial impact of stroke on primary support persons. *Psychology and Aging, 3,* 131–141.

Shanas, E. (1979). The family as a social support system in old age. *The Gerontologist, 19,* 169–174.

Shanas, E., & Maddox, G. L. (1985). Health, health resources and the utilization of care. In R. H. Binstock & E. Shanas (Eds.), *Handbook of aging and the social sciences,* (2nd ed., pp. 696–726). New York: Van Nostrand Reinhold.

Shapiro, J. P. (1992). The elderly are not children. *U.S. News & World Report,* January 13, 26–28.

Shaver, P., Furman, W., & Buhrmester, D. (1985). Transition to college: Network changes, social skills, and loneliness. In S. Duck & D. Perlman (Eds.), *Understanding personal relationships: An interdisciplinary approach* (pp. 193–219). Beverly Hills: Sage.

Sheehan, N. W. (1986). Informal support among the elderly in public senior housing. *The Gerontologist, 26,* 171–175.

Sheehan, N. W. (1989). The Caregiver Information Project: A mechanism to assist religious leaders to help family caregivers. *The Gerontologist, 29,* 703–706.

Shulman, M. D., & Mandel, E. (1988). Communication training of relatives and friends of institutionalized elderly persons. *The Gerontologist, 28,* 797–799.

Silverstein, M., & Bengtson, V. L. (1991). Do close parent–child relations reduce the mortality risk of older parents? *Journal of Health and Social Behavior, 32,* 382–395.

Skaff, M. M., & Pearlin, L. I. (1992). Caregiving: Role engulfment and the loss of self. *The Gerontologist, 32,* 656–664.

Smeeding, T. M. (1990). Economic status of the elderly. In R. H. Binstock & L. K. George (Eds.). *Handbook of aging and the social sciences* (3rd ed., pp. 362–381). San Diego: Academic Press.

Smith, T. W. (1992). Hostility and health: Current status of a psychosomatic hypothesis. *Health Psychology, 11,* 139–150.

Smyer, M. A., Zarit, S. H., & Qualls, S. H. (1990). Psychological intervention with the aging individual. In J. E. Birren & K. W. Schaie (Eds.), *Handbook of the psychology of aging* (3rd ed., pp. 375–403). San Diego: Academic Press.

Spence, J. T. (1983). Comment on Lubinski, Tellegen, and Butcher's "Masculinity, femininity, and androgyny viewed and assessed as distinct concepts." *Journal of Personality and Social Psychology, 44,* 440–446.

Spirduso, W. W., & MacRae, P. G. (1990). Motor performance and aging. In J. E. Birren & K. W. Schaie (Eds.), *Handbook of the psychology of aging* (3rd ed., pp. 183–200). San Diego: Academic Press.

Spitzberg, B. H., & Cupach, W. R. (1989). *Handbook of interpersonal competence research.* New York: Springer-Verlag.

Spitzberg, B. H., & Hecht, M. L. (1984). A component model of relational competence. *Human Communication Research, 10,* 575–599.

Stack, C. (1975). *All our kin: Strategies for survival in a black community.* New York: Harper & Row.

Steinbach, U. (1992). Social networks, institutionalization, and mortality among elderly people in the United States. *Journal of Gerontology: Social Sciences, 47,* S183–S190.

Stephens, M. A. P. (1990). Social relationships as coping resources in later-life families. In M. A. P. Stephens, J. H. Crowther, S. E. Hobfoll, & D. L. Tennenbaum (Eds.), *Stress and coping in later-life families* (pp. 1–20). New York: Hemisphere.

Stephens, M. A. P., & Bernstein, M. D. (1984). Social support and well-being among residents of planned housing. *The Gerontologist, 24,* 144–148.

Stephens, M. A. P., Crowther, J. H., Hobfoll, S. E., & Tennenbaum, D. L. (Eds.). (1990). *Stress and coping in later-life families.* New York: Hemisphere.

Stephens, M. A. P., & Hobfoll, S. E. (1990). Ecological perspectives on stress and coping in later-life families. In M. A. P. Stephens, J. H. Crowther, S. E. Hobfoll, & D. L. Tennenbaum (Eds.), *Stress and coping in later-life families* (pp. 287–304). New York: Hemisphere.

Stephens, M. A. P., Kinney, J. M., Ritchie, S. W., & Norris, V. K. (1987). Social networks as assets and liabilities in recovery from stroke by geriatric patients. *Psychology and Aging, 2,* 125–129.

Sternberg, R. J. (1990). *Wisdom: Its nature, origins, and development.* Cambridge, England: Cambridge University Press.

Sterns, H. L. (1986). Training and retraining adult and older adult workers. In J. E. Birren, P. K. Robinson, & J. E. Livingston (Eds.), *Age, health, and employment* (pp. 93–113). Englewood Cliffs, NJ: Prentice-Hall.

Sterns, H. L., Barrett, G. V., & Alexander, R. A. (1985). Accidents and the aging individual. In J. E. Birren & K. W. Schaie (Eds.), *Handbook of the psychology of aging* (2nd ed., pp. 703–724). New York: Van Nostrand Reinhold.

Stone, R., Cafferata, G. L., & Sangel, J. (1987). Caregivers of the frail elderly: A national profile. *The Gerontologist, 27,* 616–626.

Stroebe, M. S., & Stroebe, W. (1993). The mortality of bereavement: A review. In M. S. Stroebe, W. Stroebe, & R. O. Hansson (Eds.), *Handbook of bereavement: Theory, research, and intervention* (pp. 175–195). Cambridge, England: Cambridge University Press.

Stroebe, M. S., Stroebe, W., & Hansson, R. O. (Eds.). (1993). *The handbook of bereavement.* New York: Cambridge University Press.

Stroebe, W., & Stroebe, M. S. (1987). *Bereavement and health.* New York: Cambridge University Press.

Stroebe, W., & Stroebe, M. S. (1993). Determinants of adjustment to bereavement in young widows and widowers. In M. S. Stroebe, W. Stroebe, & R. Hansson (Eds.), *The handbook of bereavement* (pp. 208–226). New York: Cambridge University Press.

Sussman, M. B. (1985). The family life of old people. In R. H. Binstock & E.

Shanas (Eds.), *Handbook of aging and the social sciences* (2nd ed., pp. 415–449). New York: Van Nostrand Reinhold.

Talbott, M. M. (1990). The negative side of the relationship between older widows and their adult children: The mothers' perspective. *The Gerontologist, 30,* 595–603.

Tesch, S. A., Nehrke, M. F., & Whitbourne, S. K. (1989). Social relationships, psychosocial adaptation, and intrainstitutional relocation of elderly men. *The Gerontologist, 29,* 517–523.

Thoits, P. A. (1982). Conceptual, methodological, and theoretical problems in studying social support as a buffer against life stress. *Journal of Health and Social Behavior, 23,* 145–159.

Thomas, P. D., Goodwin, J. M., & Goodwin, J. S. (1985). Effect of social support on stress-related changes in cholesterol level, uric acid, and immune function in an elderly sample. *American Journal of Psychiatry, 142,* 735–737.

Thompson, L. W., Gallagher, D. E., & Breckenridge, J. S. (1987). Comparative effectiveness of psychotherapies for depressed elders. *Journal of Consulting and Clinical Psychology, 55,* 385–390.

Thompson, M. G., & Heller, K. (1990). Facets of support related to well-being: Quantitative social isolation and perceived family support in a sample of elderly women. *Psychology and Aging, 5,* 535–544.

Thompson, S. C. (1991). Intervening to enhance perceptions of control. In C. R. Snyder & D. R. Forsyth (Eds.), *Handbook of social and clinical psychology: The health perspective* (pp. 607–623). New York: Pergamon.

Thorndike, R. L. (1920). Intelligence and its uses. *Harpers Monthly, 140,* 227–235.

Timko, C., & Moos, R. H. (1990). Determinants of interpersonal support and self-direction in group residential facilities. *Journal of Gerontology: Social Sciences, 45,* S184–S192.

Tizard, B., & Tizard, J. A. (1970). The cognitive development of young children in residential care. *Journal of Child Psychology and Psychiatry, 11,* 177–186.

Toseland, R. W., Rossiter, C. M., Peak, T., & Smith, G. C. (1990). Comparative effectiveness of individual and group interventions to support family caregivers. *Social Work, 35,* 209–217.

Trapnell, P. D., & Wiggins, J. S. (1990). Extension of the Interpersonal Adjective Scales to include the Big Five dimensions of personality. *Journal of Personality and Social Psychology, 59,* 781–790.

Troll, L. E. (1988). New thoughts on old families. *The Gerontologist, 28,* 586–591.

U.S. Bureau of the Census. (1984a). *Current population reports* (Series P-23, No. 138): *Demographic and socioeconomic aspects of aging in the United States.* Washington, DC: U.S. Government Printing Office.

U.S. Bureau of the Census. (1984b). *Marital status and living arrangements: Current population reports, March 1982.* Washington, DC: U.S. Government Printing Office.

U.S. Bureau of the Census. (1988). Money income and poverty status in the

United States, 1987. *Current population reports* (Series P-60, No. 161, August). Washington, DC: U.S. Government Printing Office.

U.S. Bureau of the Census. (1990). *Statistical Abstract of the United States: 1990* (110th ed.). Washington, DC: U.S. Government Printing Office.

U.S. Congress, House Select Committee on Aging. (1980). *Elder abuse: The hidden problem*. Washington, DC: U.S. Government Printing Office.

U.S. Congress, House Select Committee on Aging. (1987). *Abuses in guardianship of the elderly and infirm: A national disgrace*. 100th Congress, First Session (Comm. Pub. No. 100-641). Washington, DC: U.S. Government Printing Office.

U.S. Congress, House Ways and Means Committee. (1988). *Background material and data on programs within the jurisdiction of the House Ways and Means Committee*. Washington, DC: U.S. Government Printing Office.

U.S. Department of Health and Human Services. (1991). *Healthy people 2000: National health promotion and disease prevention objectives*. DHHS Publication No. (PHS) 91-50213. Washington, DC: U.S. Government Printing Office.

Vachon, M. L. S., & Stylianos, S. K. (1988). The role of social support in bereavement. *Journal of Social Issues, 44,* 175–190.

Van Wylen, M. D., & Dykema-Lamse, J. (1990). Feelings group for adult day care. *The Gerontologist, 30,* 557–559.

Vitaliano, P. P., Russo, J., Young, H. M., Teri, L., & Maiuro, R. D. (1991). Predictors of burden in spouse caregivers of individuals with Alzheimer's disease. *Psychology and Aging, 6,* 392–402.

Waitzkin, H., & Stoeckle, J. D. (1976). Information control and micropolitics of health care: Summary of an ongoing research project. *Social Science and Medicine, 10,* 263–276.

Walker, A. J., Martin, S. S. K., & Jones, L. L. (1992). The benefits and costs of caregiving and care receiving for daughters and mothers. *Journal of Gerontology: Social Sciences, 47,* S130–S139.

Watson, D., Clark, L. A., McIntyre, C. W., & Hamaker, S. (1992). Affect, personality, and social activity. *Journal of Personality and Social Psychology, 63,* 1011–1025.

Waxler-Morrison, N., Hislop, T. G., Mears, B., & Can, L. (1991). The facts on social relationships on survival with women with breast cancer: A prospective study. *Social Science and Medicine, 33,* 177–183.

Weiss, R. S. (1974). The provisions of social relationships. In Z. Rubin (Ed.), *Doing unto others* (pp. 17–26). Englewood Cliffs, NJ: Prentice-Hall.

Weiss, R. S. (1988). Loss and recovery. *Journal of Social Issues, 44,* 37–52.

Welin, L., Svardsudd, K., Ander-Peciva, S., Tibblin, G., Tibblin, B., & Larsson, G. (1985). Prospective study of social influences on mortality. *Lancet, 2,* 915–918.

Wells, L., & Macdonald, G. (1981). Interpersonal networks and post-relocation adjustment of the institutionalized elderly. *The Gerontologist, 21,* 177–183.

Wiggins, J. S. (1973). *Personality and prediction: Principles of personality assessment*. Reading, MA: Addison-Wesley.

Wiggins, J. S. (1982). Circumplex models of interpersonal behavior in clinical psychology. In P. C. Kendall & J. N. Butcher (Eds.), *Handbook of research methods in clinical psychology* (pp. 183–221). New York: Wiley.

Wiggins, J. S., & Broughton, R. (1984). The interpersonal circle: A structural model for the integration of personality research. In R. Hogan & W. H. Jones (Eds.), *Perspectives in personality: Theory, measurement, and interpersonal dynamics* (Vol. 1, pp. 1–47). Greenwich, CT: JAI Press.

Wiggins, J. S., Trapnell, P., & Phillips, N. (1988). Psychometric and geometric characteristics of the revised Interpersonal Adjective Scales (IAS-R). *Multivariate Behavioral Research, 23,* 517–530.

Wilber, K. H. (1991). Alternatives to conservatorship: The role of daily money management services. *The Gerontologist, 31,* 150–155.

Williamson, G. M., & Schulz, R. (1990). Relationship orientation, quality of prior relationship, and distress among caregivers of Alzheimer's patients. *Psychology and Aging, 5,* 502–509.

Williamson, G. M., & Schulz, R. (1992). Physical illness and symptoms of depression among elderly outpatients. *Psychology and Aging, 7,* 343–351.

Willie, C. V. (1988). *A new look at black families.* Dix Hills, NY: General Hall.

Willis, S. L. (1985). Towards an educational psychology of the older adult learner: Intellectual and cognitive bases. In J. E. Birren & K. W. Schaie (Eds.), *Handbook of the psychology of aging* (2nd ed., pp. 818–847). New York: Van Nostrand Reinhold.

Willis, S. L. (1987). Cognitive training and everyday competence. *Annual Review of Gerontology and Geriatrics, 7,* 159–188.

Winstead, B. A., Derlega, V. J., Lewis, R. J., Margulis, S. T. (1988). Understanding the therapeutic relationship as a personal relationship. *Journal of Social and Personal Relationships, 5,* 109–125.

Wolinski, M. A. (1986). Marital therapy with older couples. *Casework: The Journal of Contemporary Social Work, 67,* 475–483.

Wolinsky, F. D., & Johnson, R. J. (1992). Widowhood, health status, and the use of health services by older adults: A cross-sectional and prospective approach. *Journal of Gerontology: Social Sciences, 47,* S95–S101.

Wortman, C. B., Silver, R. C., & Kessler, R. C. (1993). The meaning of loss and adjustment to bereavement. In M. S. Stroebe, W. Stroebe, & R. O. Hansson (Eds.), *Handbook of bereavement* (pp. 349–366). New York: Cambridge University Press.

Wrightsman, L. (1964). Measurement of philosophies of human nature. *Psychological Reports, 14,* 743–751.

Yeatts, A. (1993). *Problems in mentoring relationships.* Unpublished doctoral dissertation, The University of Tulsa.

Zarit, S. II. (1990). Interventions with frail elders and their families: Are they effective and why? In M. A. P. Stephens, J. H. Crowther, S. E. Hobfoll, & D. L. Tennenbaum (Eds.), *Stress and coping in later-life families* (pp. 241–265). Washington DC: Hemisphere.

Zarit, S. H., Birkel, R. C., & Malone Beach, E. (1989). Spouses as caregivers: Stresses and interventions. In M. Z. Goldstein (Ed.), *Family involvement in the treatment of the frail elderly.* Washington, DC: American Psychiatric Association.

Author Index

Subject Index